AF606848

IMPROVE YOUR GUT HEALTH

pil
Publications International, Ltd.

Louis Weber, CEO
Publications International, Ltd.
8140 Lehigh Ave
Morton Grove, IL 60053

Pictured on the front cover: Chicken and Fruit Salad *(page 106).*

Pictured on the back cover *(clockwise from top right):* Tofu “Fried” Rice *(page 121),* Toasted Coconut Quinoa Balls *(page 174)* and Szechuan Grilled Flank Steak *(page 84).*

Contributing Writer: Jacqueline B Marcus, MS, RDN, LDN, CNS, FADA, FAND

ISBN: 978-1-63938-546-1

Manufactured in China.

8 7 6 5 4 3 2 1

Microwave Cooking: Microwave ovens vary in wattage. Use the cooking times as guidelines and check for doneness before adding more time.

Note: This publication is only intended to provide general information. The information is specifically not intended to be a substitute for medical diagnosis or treatment by your physician or other health care professional. You should always consult your own physician or other health care professionals about any medical questions, diagnosis, or treatment. (Products vary among manufacturers. Please check labels carefully to confirm nutritional values.)

The information obtained by you from this book should not be relied upon for any personal, nutritional, or medical decision. You should consult an appropriate professional for specific advice tailored to your specific situation. PIL makes no representations or warranties, express or implied, with respect to your use of this information.

In no event shall PIL, its affiliates or advertisers be liable for any direct, indirect, punitive, incidental, special, or consequential damages, or any damages whatsoever including, without limitation, damages for personal injury, death, damage to property, or loss of profits, arising out of or in any way connected with the use of any of the above-referenced information or otherwise arising out of the use of this book.

Let’s get social!

 @Publications_International

 @PublicationsInternational

www.pilbooks.com

TABLE OF CONTENTS

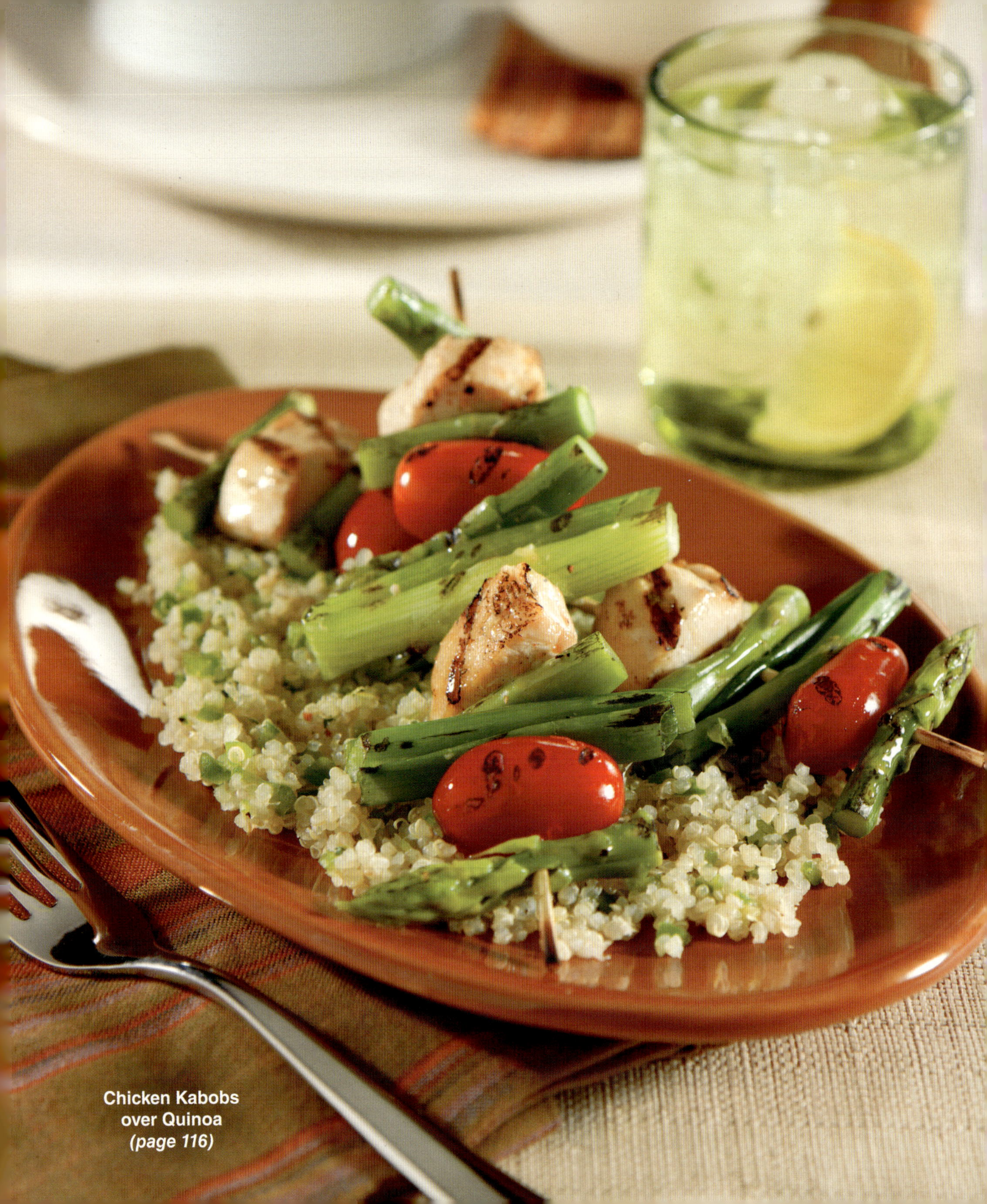

Chicken Kabobs over Quinoa *(page 116)*

INTRODUCTION

Eating and drinking are often taken for granted. Normally the human body's digestive system digests and metabolizes everything we eat and drink for energy or storage and the rest is eliminated. That is, unless there are snags along the pathway such as food allergies, intolerances or sensitivities, or a problematic gastrointestinal (GI) tract.

By understanding what happens to every mouthful, you may be able to appreciate your next bite or swallow and think about how to treat your GI tract (aka "gut") for maximal performance and health.

Good nutrition begins and depends upon effective digestion, absorption, and metabolism of nutrients. For people with gut problems, you'll find clarity in how to manage GI disorders for better nutrition and health.

Digestion and Gut Health

Digestion is the process by which foods and beverages are physically and chemically altered into smaller components by the human body that are then absorbed, metabolized for energy, or stored for future use.

During each stage of the digestive process (oral cavity, stomach, small, and large intestines), the macronutrients carbohydrates, fats, and proteins are broken down into their building blocks.

Along with vitamins, minerals, and water, these building blocks are used to fuel the body, build or rebuild it, protect the body from disease, rebound from illnesses, and a host of other functions.

What is not utilized is stored in forms that the body may be able to tap if and when necessary. All of these functions depend upon healthy digestion.

Sensory Stimuli

Digestion is activated by reactions to sensory stimuli. *Sensory stimuli* (how foods and beverages look, smell, and even sound) inform and protect the human body and trigger digestive juices "to flow."

Foods or beverages that are perceived as tasty may pleasantly stimulate the central nervous system, while foods or beverages that are perceived as offensive may have adverse effects.

Then chemical messengers in the oral cavity and GI tract transmit this information to the brain that triggers salivation and readies the body for digestion.

Normal Digestion

Normal digestion may take from 24 to 48, even up to 72 hours depending upon the composition of foods and beverages.

By and large, the more components of a food or beverage, the more challenging it is for the body to handle. Carbohydrates tend to take the shortest amount of time for digestion (sugars in soft drinks may take as little as 15 minutes, and starches in pasta may take upwards of 2 to 3 hours).

A skinless chicken breast may take 5 to 6 hours to fully digest its protein, a cup of fruit juice may digest faster than a piece of fruit because of its higher fiber composition, and butter with its saturated fat content may need about 9 to 12 hours to complete digestion.

Oral Cavity

Chemical and physical digestion starts in the *oral cavity.* The oral cavity includes the lips, inside lining of the lips and cheeks, teeth, gums, front two-thirds of the tongue, floor of the mouth below the tongue, and the bony roof of the mouth.

In *chemical digestion,* digestive enzymes such as *salivary amylase* are released by the salivary glands to begin the chemical digestive process. In *physical digestion* the teeth and tongue help to break down, moisten, and move foods to the back of the oral cavity for swallowing.

When foods are mixed with saliva they form a *bolus*, or ball that is propelled backward via the tongue for swallowing into the *esophagus*, a short tube that is lined with saliva for moisture and protection. A cartilage flap covers the esophagus that prevents the bolus from entering the *trachea* or windpipe.

The esophagus is actually a band of strong muscles that pump and propel food to the stomach. At the end of the esophagus is the cardiac sphincter, a valve that closes the opening once the bolus enters the stomach.

If the cardiac sphincter does not operate properly, then foods and beverages may back up from the stomach and cause acid reflux that may be controlled by a number of factors such as diet, medications, smaller meals, or surgery.

Stomach

Once inside the stomach, stomach enzymes, along with *hydrochloric acid* (a strong acid that digests proteins) and mucous, break down foods and beverages that contain proteins. Muscular contractions then help to convert the bolus into *chyme*, a semifluid of partially digested foods and gastric fluids.

Carbohydrates and fats are fairly undigested in the stomach; they move into the small intestine for additional digestion.

Small Intestine

The small intestine is small in diameter but long in uncoiled length (about 20 to 23 feet in total and about one inch in diameter). It contains three sections: the *duodenum*, *jejunum* and *ileum*. Together they work with the *gallbladder*, *liver*, and *pancreas*—three organs that secrete substances into the small intestine that continue to digest chyme.

The *duodenum* is short; it prepares the absorption of nutrients by mixing chyme from the stomach, digestive fluids from the pancreas, and bile from the liver. The *jejunum* is located in the midsection of the small intestine where the products of nutrient digestion (amino acids, fatty acids, and sugars) are absorbed. The *ileum* mainly absorbs bile acids, vitamin B12, and other remaining nutrients.

The *gallbladder* secretes *bile* (an emulsifier that contains cholesterol) into the small intestine to help digest fats. The *liver* detoxifies metabolites, participates in metabolism, produces biochemicals for digestion, regulates glycogen storage, and synthesizes proteins among many other functions. The liver also produces bile that is stored in the gallbladder. This is why the liver is so vital.

The *pancreas* also secretes substances into the small intestine for digestion. Pancreatic secretions help to neutralize acidic chyme from the stomach and its digestive enzymes help to further digest carbohydrates, fats, and proteins respectively.

The pancreas produces *insulin* and *glucagon*, two important *hormones* essential in carbohydrate metabolism for maintaining blood glucose (sugar). Insulin is secreted by the beta cells of the pancreas to handle elevated blood glucose, while alpha cells of the pancreas secrete glucagon in response to low blood glucose. The pancreas is also a very critical body organ.

Large Intestine

The *large intestine* is shorter in length (about 5 feet) but larger in diameter (about 3 inches) than the small intestine. It contains the *cecum*, *colon*, and *rectum*.

What is not absorbed by the small intestine moves into the large intestine and blends with water and minerals. There is some vitamin absorption, but essentially the main functions of the large intestine are to hold and help excrete the remains of digested foods and beverages via its strong muscles.

Factors That Affect Healthy Digestion

An intact and fully functional digestive tract provides the framework for healthy digestion and metabolism. Activity level, conditions and diseases, diet, genes, medications, stress, and other factors may affect healthy digestion.

Good vs. Bad Bacteria

Bacteria, *fungi*, and *viruses* are miniscule microbes that reside in the intestines as well as inside the genitalia, mouth, nose, urinary tract, and on the skin. A microbiome is a collection of these microbes that is unique for each individual. It is determined by genetics and lifestyle among other factors.

In the bigger picture, microbiome disruption and/or bacteria imbalances may be associated with conditions or diseases such as colon cancer, diabetes, and obesity. Microbiome bacteria imbalances may also contribute to *inflammatory autoimmune diseases* such as inflammatory bowel disease including Crohn's disease, lupus, and rheumatoid arthritis.

Modifying one's microbiome through environmental and lifestyle changes may provide some insights into these diseases and others and outline courses of action.

Healthy Gut Flora

Since gut bacteria line the intestines, they are involved with the digestion and absorption of foods and beverages. Gut bacteria also help communicate with the body's immune system, influence brain functioning, and produce vitamins that are necessary for life.

It's possible that people with GI conditions and diseases have different compositions of gut bacteria that affect these functions and others. It may also be that a *diversity* of gut bacteria is more important than the presence or absence of specific gut bacteria.

Imbalanced gut bacteria may also be linked with attention-deficit-disorder, anxiety, autism, Alzheimer's disease, cardiovascular disease, and depression. This is because gut bacteria may be able to produce *metabolites*, or small molecules than may make their way to the brain, heart, and other organs and affect their normal functioning.

Improving Gut Flora

Gut flora may improve with a diet that is lower in fats and sugars and higher in certain fibers. By making certain dietary changes, a person may be able to alter their microbiome, improve their immune function, reduce inflammation, and be healthier overall. Drinking more water, managing stress, and incorporating exercise into daily activities may also help support a healthier microbiome.

Healthy gut bacteria may be increased through the addition of *fermented foods* with *probiotics*, live bacteria and yeasts that include certain types of yogurt, kefir (a yogurt-based beverage), miso, pickles, and sauerkraut. Another option is the use of *probiotic supplements* with similar functionality. Probiotic supplements are thought to be safe but they may have side effects and/or trigger allergic reactions.

People with depressed immune function due to chemotherapy or late-stage cancer should be cautioned about taking probiotic supplements since they may be incompatible with treatments.

Digestive Disorders

When a finely tuned digestive system becomes misaligned, a host of GI disorders and systemic issues may arise that may affect a number of other bodily functions.

Digestive disorders from simple stomach pains to more complicated diseases, such as celiac disease or gluten intolerance, may impact this very intricate yet naturally ongoing biological process of digestion. This may be due to bacteria and/or enzyme disorders, stomach acid imbalances, inflammation, and other states.

Symptoms

Common symptoms of GI disorders may include any or many of the following conditions: abdominal pain/syndrome, acid reflux, belching, biliary tract disorders, bloating, constipation, dyspepsia, flatulence (gas), gallbladder disorders, gallstone pancreatitis, gastro-esophageal reflux disease, heartburn, hemorrhoids, indigestion, irritable bowel syndrome, nausea, peptic ulcer disease, vomiting, and more.

Identification

Imaging tests such as abdominal ultrasound, abdominal X-ray, computed tomography (CT) scan, CT angiography, magnetic resonance imaging (MRI), radionuclide scanning, virtual colonoscopy, and upper and lower GI tests may be used to detect GI irregularities.

Upper GI tests may be used to examine the esophagus, stomach, and duodenum and to diagnose esophageal variances, hiatal hernias, obstruction, or narrowing of the upper GI tract, tumors, ulcers, and other anomalies.

Lower GI tests may be used to detect Crohn's disease, colon polyps, diverticular disease, gastroenteritis, strictures or site narrowing and/or obstruction, tumors, ulcerative colitis, and more.

Body awareness may be the first identification of GI disorders and defense. Regular medical examinations may detect underlying symptoms.

Food Allergies, Intolerances, and Sensitivities

An *allergy* is an immune system disorder. A food allergy or *hypersensitivity* is a reaction to a substance in a food or beverage.

An allergic food reaction occurs when a substance in the environment that is known as an allergen prompts an allergic reaction by the human body. Common allergic reactions to foods and beverages may include asthma, eczema, hay fever, hives, and GI reactions.

In contrast, *food intolerance* is hypersensitivity to a non-allergic food or beverage. By and large, food intolerance does not provoke an abnormal response to the proteins in foods and beverages, though some of the symptoms may be similar. These may include aches and pains, bloating, cramping, diarrhea, headaches, heartburn, irritability, nausea, stomach pain, and/or vomiting.

In general, food intolerances are more common than diagnosed food allergies. For example, gluten and lactose intolerance are considered food intolerances, not allergies since they may not be triggered by the immune system nor life-threatening.

In general, the removal of suspected foods and beverages that are connected with food intolerances may be effective for remedying symptoms.

The term *food sensitivity* is sometimes used interchangeably with food intolerance. Food sensitivities imply that there are sensitive reactions to food, rather than intolerance that may be mild, not immediate nor life-threatening.

Food sensitivities may be mainly digestive in nature and may not become evident for some time after a suspected food or beverage is consumed.

Gluten Intolerance and Sensitivity

Gluten intolerance is the inability of the human body to tolerate the protein gluten. Gluten intolerance is different from a wheat allergy in that it is a severe and sudden response to wheat.

Gluten intolerance is actually due to *gliaden*, a component of gluten that is responsible for the action of bread to rise. Gliaden prompts the autoimmune system to react to the tissues in the small intestine and produce an inflammatory response. The *villi* (small hair-like projections that protrude from the intestinal wall) become flattened and unable to assist nutrient transport and absorption into the bloodstream. This may be detected by biopsies or blood tests.

Many foods and beverages contain gluten that is obvious, hidden, or sometimes unexpected. Gluten may be found in common and ancient grains that include barley, brewer's yeast, bulgur, couscous, kasha, malt (including malt extract, malt flavoring, malt syrup, malt vinegar, malted barley flour and malted milk, or milkshakes), matzo meal, oats, rye, triticale, and wheat and its varieties and derivatives (such as durum, einkorn, emmer, farina, farro, graham, kamut, semolina, spelt, and wheat berries).

Other substances in foods and beverages that may contain gluten include artificial and natural flavorings, hydrolyzed plant or vegetable proteins, and modified food starches that may be found in beer, cold cuts, egg substitutes, frozen yogurt and yogurt drinks, salad dressings, and other foods.

Tolerated grains may include corn, millet, quinoa, rice, sorghum and teff. Amaranth and pure buckwheat may also be tolerated since they are botanically considered as grains. Root and legume starches (such as arrowroot, pea, potato, or soybean) may be used in combination with tolerated grains to replicate the action of wheat-based products.

Celiac Disease

In the larger picture, gluten intolerance is considered a symptom of *celiac disease,* an autoimmune disorder of predisposed people that affects the GI tract. Symptoms of celiac disease may include anemia, diarrhea, fatigue, and/or weight loss. If damage to the small intestine occurs, then lactose intolerance may result.

Celiac disease may lead to deficiencies in vitamins A, D, E and K, folic acid, vitamin B12, calcium, and iron and generate to abdominal bleeding, anemia, and/or osteoporosis.

In comparison, *non-celiac gluten sensitivity (NCGS)* is a susceptibility to gluten in foods, beverages, and ingredients. It is not diagnosed food intolerance. NCGS is characterized by intestinal and other bodily symptoms that are related to the ingestion of foods and beverages with gluten.

By adhering to a gluten-free diet, the small intestine may be able heal and symptoms may subside, but there is no known cure for celiac disease.

Irritable Bowel Syndrome

Irritable bowel syndrome (IBS) is a common functional disorder of the GI tract that may produce abdominal pain, bloating, change in bowel habits, constipation, diarrhea, and/or gas. IBS is often included in the spectrum of gluten-related disorders along with celiac disease, non-celiac gluten sensitivity, and wheat allergy. IBS is unlike *inflammatory bowel disease* in that there is not inflammation, ulcers, or damage to the bowel.

The diagnosis of IBS is based on clinical characteristics. Alterations in intestinal motility, permeability, nutrient absorption, and intestinal microbiota (gut flora) may be indicated. Anorexia, fever, GI bleeding, and/or severe weight loss may signify a more acute situation.

Contributing factors that may lead to IBS may include alterations in brain-gut signaling, changes in the gut microbiome, genetics, impaired gut barrier functions, immune dysfunction, and psychosocial factors.

Trigger foods and beverages, particularly ones that evoke hypersensitivity to food antigens, are also implied as is accelerated colonic transit.

Dietary modifications that address IBS include the reduction of gas-producing foods such as *Fermentable Oligo-*, *Di-* and *Monosaccharides and Polyols,* (referred to as FODMAPs), gluten, and lactose.

Dietary and other approaches to IBS include an elimination diet, high and low-fiber diet, low-fat diet, gluten-free and lactose-free diets, and low-FODMAP diet in addition to decreased caffeine, increased water consumption, regular exercise, and mindfulness training.

Crohn's Disease

Crohn's disease is a chronic inflammatory disease characterized by inflammation of the GI tract. While Crohn's disease may affect any part of the GI tract from the mouth to the anus, it most often affects the small intestine. Crohn's disease may also affect the eyes, joints, and skin.

Compared to *ulcerative colitis* (another inflammatory bowel disease), Crohn's disease may appear in patches, extend through the entire thickness of the bowel wall, and have a high rate of relapse. What makes Crohn's disease different and potentially more serious than irritable bowel syndrome is its chronic inflammation.

Lactose Intolerance, Sensitivity, and Milk Allergy

Lactose intolerance is the inability of the human body to digest, metabolize, and absorb the milk sugar *lactose* that is found in some dairy milk and milk products. There is a higher incidence of lactose intolerance in countries and ethnicities where dairy milk and products are not commonly consumed, such as Africa, Asia, Central American, and the Middle East. Lactose intolerance may also increase with age if there is a reduction or absence of the enzyme *lactase* that is responsible for its breakdown.

Lactase (located in the lining of the small intestine) breaks down lactose into *glucose* and *galactose*, two simple sugars to be metabolized for energy. With insufficient lactase, lactose may collect in the small intestine since it may not be able to pass through the villi into the bloodstream. Instead, lactose may accumulate and be metabolized by intestinal bacteria that may cause fermentation and a range of symptoms. These may include bloating, cramping, diarrhea, or gas.

A heightened reaction to lactose may be detected by a blood sugar test, elimination of dairy products, hydrogen breath test, physical exam, or stool sample.

Lactose sensitivity may not clearly be detected as reactions may be sporadic. *Milk allergy* is an allergic response that involves the immune system to the protein (usually casein or whey) in milk.

Human milk is high in lactose. Buffalo, cow, goat, sheep, and yak milk contain about equal amounts of lactose that is about one-half that of human milk. Some dairy products and butters that are fat-free or reduced in fat tend to have milk solids added, so they may be higher in lactose.

Products with less lactose include some hard cheeses, such as Parmesan, fermented cheeses such as cottage cheese, soft cheeses such as ricotta, and ice cream. Buttermilk, sour cream, and yogurt may contain some lactase that is produced by bacteria during their manufacture.

Food additives with lactose may include lactoserum, margarine, milk solids, modified milk ingredients, and whey that may be found in nondairy foods that include processed breads, meal-replacement products, and some meats.

Lactose drops and tablets may be taken before dairy products are consumed to aid their digestion. But the best strategy is avoidance. Bean, grain, and nut "milks" and some modified dairy-alternative products are available. They should be fortified with the nutrients that dairy products normally provide, especially calcium and vitamins A and D.

Leaky Gut Syndrome

Leaky gut syndrome may be more of a collection of symptoms than a diagnosed medical condition. A diagnosis of "leaky gut" may be difficult to establish due to the complexities of the gut and its immunological implications. Symptoms of "leaky gut syndrome" (as increased intestinal permeability) may appear as bloating, cramps, food sensitivities, gas, and general aches and pains.

Increased intestinal permeability is thought to be a possible cause of leaky gut syndrome. Tight junctions in the gut that control what passes through the small intestine may work improperly and permit substances to leak into the bloodstream. This condition may trigger inflammation and changes in gut flora that may lead to digestive changes and complications.

Some people who have celiac or Crohn's disease may experience leaky gut, but little more is known. The standard American diet that is low in fiber and high in saturated fats and sugars may likely play a role along with chronic stress, heavy alcohol use, and lifestyle. Some people may have a genetic predisposition.

Leaky gut may be associated with other autoimmune diseases and conditions such as acne, allergies, arthritis, asthma, chronic fatigue syndrome, fibromyalgia, lupus, mental illness, multiple sclerosis, obesity, and/or type 1 diabetes, but clinical studies do not demonstrate cause and effect. A nutritious whole foods diet with foods and beverages that help to suppress inflammation and the avoidance of those that promote inflammation may be the most defensive.

FODMAPs

FODMAPs (Fermentable Oligosaccharides, Disaccharides, Monosaccharides and Polyols) are a collection of tiny carbohydrate molecules that are naturally found in some foods in the human diet. FODMAPs may be poorly digested and absorbed by some individuals and may reach the end of the intestine where some gut bacteria reside. These bacteria may feed on FODMAPs and produce hydrogen gas, rather than methane gas that is produced by friendly bacteria.

As a result, some digestive symptoms such as bloating, constipation, diarrhea, distention, gas, and/or stomach pain may result. In particular, FODMAPs tend to be "osmotically active" which means that they may pull water into the intestine and contribute to bloating and diarrhea.

During the digestive process, when carbohydrates (starches and sugars) are broken down into their components, some are considered "short-chain" with only a few sugar molecules linked together. These include *fructose*, *fructans*, *galactans*, *lactose,* and *polyols*.

Fructose is a sugar that is naturally found in some fruits and vegetables and in "added sugars." *Fructans* are found in gluten-containing grains such as barley, rye, and wheat. *Galactans* are present in legumes. *Lactose* is found in dairy products and *polyols* appear in sugar alcohols such as *sorbitol*, *mannitol,* and *xylitol* and in some fruits and vegetables such as some apples, carrots, corn, pineapple, and plums.

A *low-FODMAP diet* is a dietary approach that may be used by some people who have *functional gastrointestinal disorders (FGID)* or irritable bowel diseases such as Crohn's disease and ulcerative colitis. A low-FODMAP diet plan limits foods, beverages, and other substances that contain foods and beverages with FODMAPs.

How the Low-FODMAP Diet Works

By eliminating foods and beverages that are high-FODMAPs and focusing on those that are low-FODMAPs, gastrointestinal symptoms may be reduced or eliminated. The more diligent that a person is in eliminating high-FODMAPs, then the more relief that they may experience.

However, instead of eliminating all high-FODMAPs, it is possible to eliminate one suspected food or beverage and observe any reactions before reintroducing or avoiding that food or beverage. This is the basis of an elimination diet that is often used to detect suspected allergens. An elimination diet may also be used in conjunction with medical tests for fructose, gluten, or lactose intolerance to rule out specific reactions to these substances.

High-FODMAP foods and beverages to exclude or limit include:

Beverages such as beer, fruit juices, high fructose corn syrup, milk, soft drinks with high-fructose corn syrup, and soy milk.

Breads, cakes, and cookies such as breads (including sourdough), bread crumbs, cakes, cookies, and sweet breads that contain rye or wheat.

Cereals such as mixed-grain, muesli, and wheat-based.

Dairy products such as fresh or soft cheeses; frozen yogurt, ice cream, milk from dairy cows, goats, and sheep; sour cream, many yogurts; and whey protein supplements.

Fruits such as fresh apples, apricots, blackberries and boysenberries, cherries, dates, figs, pears, peaches, watermelon, applesauce, and canned fruits.

Flours and grains such as barley, bulgur, chickpea flour*, couscous, durum, kamut, lentil flour*, multigrain flour, pea flour*, rye, semolina, soy flour*, triticale, wheat bran, wheat flour, and wheat germ.

**as tolerated*

Legumes such as baked beans, canned beans that include chickpeas and kidney beans, lentils and soybeans, and fresh legumes.

Nuts and seeds such as cashews and pistachios.

Pasta and noodles such as those made with mixed grain or wheat flours.

Sweeteners such as fructose, high fructose corn syrup, honey and sugar substitutes such as maltitol, mannitol, sorbitol, and xylitol.

Vegetables such as artichokes, asparagus, beets, broccoli, Brussels sprouts, cabbage, cauliflower, fennel, garlic, mushrooms, okra, onions, leeks and shallots, and peas.

Wheat products such as many breads, biscuits, breakfast cereals, crackers, pancakes, tortillas, and waffles.

In contrast, Low-FODMAP foods and beverages to incorporate include:

Beverages such as mineral or soda water, natural spring and mineral water, and many coffees and teas.

Breads, cookies, and cakes such as corn tortillas and taco shells, plain rice cakes and crackers, and gluten-free products.

Cereals such as corn or rice-based breakfast cereals, cream of buckwheat or rice, oatmeal, and gluten-free products.

Dairy products such as ripened cheeses that include Brie and Camembert, hard cheeses that include Parmesan and Romano, and dairy-free dairy products (lactose-free milk, kefir, and yogurt).

Eggs*

Fats and oils such as butter (without milk solids), ghee, lard, and vegetable oils.

Fish*

Fruits such as bananas, blueberries, cantaloupe and other melons except watermelon, grapefruit, kiwifruit, lemons, limes, mandarins, oranges, passion fruit, raspberries, and strawberries.

Flours, grains, and starches such as arrowroot, buckwheat flour, cornmeal, cornstarch, glutinous rice, ground rice, malt, millet, oat bran, oatmeal, polenta, popcorn, potato flour, quinoa, rice, rice bran, rice flour, sago, sorghum, tapioca, wild rice, and gluten-free products.

Herbs and spices (without sweet fillers)

Meats*

Nuts and seeds such as almonds, cashews, macadamia, and pine nuts and sesame seeds and their "butters" (without sweeteners).

Pasta and noodles such as glass (mung bean) noodles, pure buckwheat soba noodles, rice noodles, and rice vermicelli.

Poultry*

Sweeteners such as maple syrup, molasses, some artificial sweeteners (other than high-FODMAP), and stevia.

Vegetables such as bok choy, carrots, celery, chives and green onions, cucumbers, eggplant, green beans, kale, leafy green lettuces, parsnips, potatoes, radishes, spinach, squash including zucchini, sweet potatoes tomatoes, turnips, water chestnuts, and yams, along with alfalfa sprouts, and the rhizome ginger root.

**without added High-FODMAP ingredients*

Understanding the Nutrition Facts Label

The *Nutrition Facts Label* found on food products was designed to aid consumers in their food and beverage selections. By checking the Nutrition Facts Label and ingredient list, a person may be able to select foods and beverages with the most nutrients and least amount of excess calories, sugars, fats, sodium, and some additives and preservatives that might be detrimental to health.

Reading and comprehending the Nutrition Facts Label and ingredient list are especially important for people with GI disorders to help avoid potential food and beverage triggers before consumption.

As you review the Nutrition Facts Label, take into account these guidelines.

To Decrease Acidity

- Look for common food acids: ascetic acid (vinegar), citric acid, fumaric acid, lactic acid, malic acid, and tartaric acid.
- Consider the pH value of foods and beverages. Generally citrus fruits and juices (grapefruits, lemons, and oranges) have a low pH. Apples, blueberries, grapes, mangoes, peaches, pineapples, plums and pomegranates also tend to be acidic, as are some black coffee, milk, and sodas.
- Balance acidity with fresh vegetables (that include aloe vera, fennel, parsley, and root vegetables such as potatoes) and other more alkaline foods and substances such as bananas, bulgur wheat, couscous, fish and seafood, ginger, oatmeal, poultry, and rice.

To Decrease Fats and Oils

- Look for these terms that indicate fats or oils in an ingredient list:

Cholesterol, fatty acids, hydrogenated or partially hydrogenated oils, lecithin, margarine, monounsaturated fatty acids, polyunsaturated fatty acids, saturated fatty acids, total fat, trans fatty acids, oils (such as canola, corn, olive, peanut, safflower, soybean, sunflower and vegetable oil), omega-3 and 6-fatty acids, solids fats (such as butter, beef fat [tallow], chicken fat, coconut oil, pork fat [lard], shortening, palm oil, and palm kernel oil.

To Decrease or Eliminate Gluten

- Look for the following ingredients that generally indicate a product contains gluten:

Barley

Brewer's yeast

Malt (such as barley malt or malt vinegar); maltodextrin may be safe to consume.

Oats (unless certified gluten-free since may cross-contaminate).

Rye

Wheat and derivatives (such as modified food starch).

- "Wheat-free" does not necessarily ensure that a product is gluten-free.

To Decrease or Eliminate Lactose

- Look for the following terms that generally indicate that a product contains the milk sugar lactose:

Butter	**Curds**	**Lactose monohydrate**	**Nonfat dry milk**
Casein	**Dried milk powder**	**Milk by-products**	**Nougat**
Caseinates	**Dry milk Solids**		**Whey**
Cheese	**Lactose**		

- Avoid products with the term "may contain milk or milk solids".
- Plant-based milk substitutes that are made from almonds, oats, rice, and soy should not contain lactose and may be tolerated. They are sometimes referred to as plant "milks".
- Baking and binding agents, lactate, lactitol (a sugar alcohol), lactic acid, lactic acid bacteria (fermented lactic acid in sauerkraut, for example), milk protein and starches, and thickening agents do not tend to contain lactose.
- Lactose may also be present in prescription and over-the-counter medications, including some calcium chews and ones that are used for gas or stomach acid.

To Decrease or Eliminate Wheat

- Look for the following terms that generally indicate a product contains wheat:
- All-purpose flour, bread made with wheat or white flour, bread crumbs, bread flour, bulgur, cereal extract, couscous, cracker meal, einkorn, emmer (farro), farina, flour, graham, gluten, kamut, malt, malt extract, matzo and matzo meal, noodles, pasta, semolina, spelt, sprouted wheat, tabbouleh, triticale, triticum, wheat berries, wheat bran, wheat germ, wheat germ oil, wheat grass, wheat starch, whole wheat bread, whole wheat flour.
- Some artificial and natural flavorings, caramel color, dextrin, food starch, gelatinized starch, modified starch, modified food starch, vegetable starch, glucose syrup, hydrolyzed vegetable protein (HVP), maltodextrin, monosodium glutamate (MSG), oats, soy sauce (also shoyu, tamari and teriyaki sauce), surimi, texturized vegetable protein, and vegetable gums may also contain wheat.
- The term "wheat" may appear in parentheses in an ingredient list or a separate "contains" statement. According to the Food Allergen Labeling and Consumer Protection Act as one of the top eight allergens, wheat must be clearly identified on a food label. Derivatives of wheat, such as "modified food starch" must also be clearly identified.

To Decrease or Eliminate FODMAPs

- Look for the following terms on food labels that generally indicate a product contains FODMAPs:
- Oligosaccharides and fructans—found in barley, cashews, chamomile tea, dates, dried figs, fennel tea, garlic, inulin (as in chicory root), leeks, legumes, nectarines, onions, oolong tea, pistachios, plums, prunes, rye, shallots, soybeans, watermelon, wheat, and white peaches.
- Disaccharides (lactose)—found in cream cheese, cottage cheese, ice cream, milk, ricotta, and yogurt.
- Monosaccharides (fructose)—found in agave, apples, asparagus, cherries, high fructose corn syrup, fresh figs, honey, Jerusalem artichokes (sun chokes), mangoes, pears, sugar snap peas, and watermelon.
- Polyols (sorbitol and mannitol)—found in apples, apricots, blackberries, cauliflower, mushrooms, nectarines, peaches, pears, plums, prunes, snow peas, sweet corn, and watermelon.

To Increase Probiotics

- Look for the following terms that generally indicate a product contains probiotics:

Buttermilk	**Kim chi**	**Some juice**	**Some yogurt**
Fermented milks	**Miso**	**Some pickles**	**Soy drinks**
Kefir	**Sauerkraut**	**Some soft cheese**	**Tempeh**

- Dietary probiotics have various forms and functions, such as acidophilus (in yogurt and other fermented foods), bifidobacterium (in some dairy products such as some cheeses and yogurt), and saccharomyces boulardii (yeast found in some probiotic supplements). It is best to investigate what's right.

To Decrease or Increase Dietary Fiber

- Many foods and ingredients are sources of dietary fiber. Look for the following terms:
- Foods with insoluble fibers: avocados, bananas, cauliflower, celery, grapes, green beans, kiwi fruit, legumes, nuts and seeds, tomatoes, zucchini, and whole grains.
- Foods with soluble fibers: apples, avocados, barley, berries, broccoli, carrots, figs, flax, Jerusalem artichokes, legumes, nuts (especially almonds), oats, onions, pears, plums, psyllium, prunes, and sweet potatoes.

Deciphering Food Additives and Preservatives

Different GI problems may require the avoidance of specific food additives or preservatives. This is especially the case for FODMAPs.

In general for lactose intolerance or sensitivity, avoid additives or preservatives that include "lactose" or "lactose monohydrate."

For gluten sensitivity or intolerance, avoid artificial food colorings, artificial sweeteners, butylated hydroxytoluene (BHT) and butylated hydroxyanisole (BHA), brominated vegetable oil (BVO) and added vegetable gums.

Some food colorings, flavor enhancers, or additives may or may not contain gluten such as caramel color, hydrolyzed plant protein, maltodextrin, maltose, modified food starch, monosodium glutamate (MSG), natural and artificial flavorings, and textured vegetable protein. It's best to check directly with food manufacturers.

Dietary Challenges and Assistance

If there are one or two GI conditions or diseases, then dietary strategies may be straightforward, such as the elimination of gluten or lactose for intolerances. Dietary approaches for multiple GI conditions or diseases may be mindboggling.

The best course of action is to discover what works best for you. Note these step-by-step strategies:

Evaluate Food/Beverage Triggers

When certain foods and/or beverages cause discomfort or pain, see if avoidance produces relief. Maybe their frequency needs to be reduced. By substituting other foods or beverages, symptoms may dissipate. This step takes trial and error.

Eliminate Food Triggers

"Trigger foods", even in tiny amounts, may elicit allergic responses, such as hives, breathing problems, GI symptoms, or even anaphylaxis (a severe allergic reaction that may impair breathing and cause shock).

For example, wheat gluten may instigate intestinal cramping, but people with a wheat allergy may have a severe allergic reaction such as asthma, hives, skin rash, or intense stomach disorders such as diarrhea, vomiting, or at worst anaphylaxis.

An *elimination diet* may be used to exclude suspected food and beverage triggers and identify potential allergic or sensitive foods and beverages. A health care provider or team should closely monitor allergic individuals who undergo an elimination diet because some substances may provoke acute reactions.

Other than an elimination diet, blood and skin tests may also help to identify problematic substances.

Determine which Foods/Beverages to Avoid, Limit, and Include

The goal of a gut-healthy diet is to eliminate certain foods and beverages that are suspected of provoking symptoms; limit others that may be intermittently tolerated, and support remaining foods and beverages for inclusion and well-being. This may vary according to individualized needs so one overall gut-healthy dietary approach may be complicated.

Evaluate Other Factors

Fiber is important for healthy digestion since it serves to push foods through the GI tract, create volume and weight to the feces to make it softer and easier to pass, and provide fullness and satisfaction.

- A fiber-rich diet has been connected to decreased incidences of certain cancers, cardiovascular disease, diabetes, and other chronic conditions and diseases. These disorders may be reduced by the inclusion of fresh fruits and vegetables, legumes, nuts and seeds, and whole grains, if tolerated.

Hydration is essential for fiber to be effective. Water is vital for many bodily functions involved in healthy digestion, including the effective use of fiber. Natural spring and mineral water are best options.

The amount of water that one consumes may lead to constipation or diarrhea. If too little water is consumed, then more salts and water are absorbed from the bowel and the chances of constipation may increase. If too much water is consumed, then this may lead to bloating or acid reflux by flushing the stomach contents into the esophagus.

- Soda and other soft drinks should be avoided since they may add carbonation, excess calories, and sugars. Pure fruit and vegetables juices may still be high in calories and sugars. Caffeinated coffees and teas may stimulate the gut. Some herbal teas might cause some sensitivities since they may cross-react with food allergens. Unsweetened dairy milk alternatives provide protein and vitamin and mineral-rich options.
- Alcoholic beverages should only be used in moderation, if tolerated, since alcohol may impair muscle function and contribute to heartburn and diarrhea, damage the musical lining of the esophagus, increase the risk of esophageal cancer, and impair nutrient absorption.

Processed foods are often higher in calories and some fats, sodium, and sugars that are counter-indicated for gut-healthy eating. When in doubt, select foods and beverages that are in their most natural states and farm-raised, grass-fed, in-season, and organic as much as possible.

Probiotics may be used to support a well-chosen gut-healthy meal plan.

Supplements may have their place in a gut-healthy diet, but a well-formulated food and beverage protocol should be constructed first and then any gaps identified and addressed.

Create a Personalized Plan for Optimal Gut Health

By taking the aforementioned strategies into account a person may be able to create a list of foods and beverages to USE, LIMIT, and AVOID for optimal gut health. With this list, foods and beverages to USE may be divided into meals and snacks. Try to include protein, healthy carbohydrates, and fats at each meal or mini-meal for optimum nutrition and satisfaction.

Journal Foods, Beverages, Exercise, Mindfulness, and Reactions

Journal writing and on-line tracking programs provide opportunities to tag certain foods and beverages, track exercise, program mindfulness, and chart physical and emotional responses. This accounting may be useful for noting which strategies work and which others may need revising.

Plan a Gut-Healthy Food Pantry

Since there is a wide array of GI conditions, an all-encompassing list of gut-health foods and beverages may not be as pinpointed as required. Instead, refer to each of the conditions to learn which foods and beverages to stock or exclude.

Cook Gut-Healthy Foods

One of the most important considerations for gut-healthy cooking is the avoidance of cross-contamination in food and beverage preparation, cooking, and clean up. Even the tiniest amounts of questionable substances may precipitate allergic or sensitivity reactions in prone individuals.

Keep preparation areas sanitized, separate trigger foods and beverages, store foods and beverages separately from non-sanctioned items, and cleanse thoroughly.

Smart cooking techniques that decrease or preserve nutrients without additional calories should be used. These include boiling, broiling, grilling, poaching, steaming, and stir-frying.

Enjoy Stress-Free Eating

Make mealtime as enjoyable as possible by practicing mindfulness and enjoying the companionship of others. For independent living, focus on slowing down, enjoying each mouthful or swallow, placing silverware down between bites, and thinking pleasant thoughts.

Eat Gut-Healthy On-the-Go

Eating and drinking gut-healthy foods and beverages may seem challenging at home; however, gut-healthy dining may be especially difficult when eating out or traveling.

Many restaurant menus are available online which makes reviewing and evaluating menus easier. If questions arise, diners may contact restaurants directly and inquire about specific ingredients and preparations.

Be proactive and inform servers about desirable/undesirable foods and beverages. When in doubt, do not order or share questionable dishes. By ordering plain foods that are simply prepared, some sensitive food triggers may be alleviated. Still, even simple protein foods may be marinated or seasoned with ingredients that precipitate adverse gut reactions.

In general, people with diagnosed allergies, intolerances, or sensitivities should limit or avoid certain restaurants where trigger substances are prominent. A "chef card" may be carried that states food and beverage restrictions. Farm-to-table menus with farm-raised, grass-fed, in-season, organic foods, and beverages may be preferred.

Other Lifestyle Choices

Practice Mindfulness

Mindfulness is the ability to focus the mind on a certain moment and accepting the significances. Mindfulness is both a preventive and therapeutic technique that helps a person to achieve a mental state where bodily sensations, feelings, and thoughts are fairly synchronized. Some people might think of mindfulness as meditation while others might view it as "seizing the moment."

Mindfulness might take backstage to the frantic pace that modern life dictates. For those with GI issues, mindfulness might be "just what the doctor ordered" for calming an over-sensitive GI tract.

The use of mindfulness to handle emotions and stresses that may directly or indirectly affect the gut has been demonstrated in patient studies. Poor gut health has also been implicated in some neurological and neuropsychiatric disorders. By taking the time to slow down, practicing deep breathing and engaging in some calming self-talk, along with a gut-healthy personalized treatment plan, some GI symptoms may be alleviated.

Keep Active

Daily activities and exercise are important for healthy lifestyles that promote mental and physical wellbeing and gut health.

Exercise helps to attain and maintain a healthy weight, enhance nutrient uptake and usage, improve circulation, strengthen the heart and lungs, and support digestion. About 30 minutes of daily exercise is recommended daily.

Regular exercise may also contribute to regular bowel habits since it stimulates the intestinal muscles to contract and push digested substances out of the large intestine through peristalsis and influence normal bowel contraction.

Seeking Additional Help

Chronic gut-related symptoms such as abdominal pain, bloody stool, excessive constipation, diarrhea, distention, gas, and/or sudden weight gain or loss may prompt immediate need for consultation by a health care provider. One that specializes in functional medicine may not only help treat the symptoms but may also try to evaluate the causes and any underlying deficiencies, excesses, or imbalances.

Some examinations and tests might be warranted that include blood chemistry analysis, Elimination Diet, food sensitivity testing, hair mineral analysis, saliva, stool and urine specimen analysis, and/or neurotransmitter profile. Not all of these procedures are considered valid or definitive on their own. They should be viewed comprehensibly for an integrative care approach.

The services of a *Registered Dietitian/Nutritionist (RDN)* may be helpful within the realm of an integrated health care team for devising an individualized gut-healthy diet plan that integrates medications and supplements, if necessary. Make sure that the RDN is a certified provider through the Academy of Nutrition and Dietetics.

Make a Gut-Healthy Lifestyle Work for You

Some people are very motivated to change their diet and lifestyle on their own while others may require major incentives and support. There are both short- and longer-term benefits for undertaking a gut-healthy approach to diet and lifestyle.

For some people, the short-term relief from distressing gastrointestinal symptoms may be encouraging. For others, the hope for longer-term protection from potentially debilitating chronic conditions and diseases may be inspiring. Even if followed to a limited extent, gut-healthy eating and drinking may offer a nutritious approach to foods and beverages, diet, and well-being.

Gut-Healthy Recipes

The following pages include more than 85 healthy and easy-to-prepare recipes that may work for you. Take note of your specific condition, whether it is a food intolerance or sensitivity, irritable bowel, leaky gut, or other digestive disorder, and select those recipes with ingredients that are best tolerated. Make modifications, as necessary, that allow these recipes to fit your particular needs.

These recipes were collected with the various "gut" conditions in mind, and given that different foods and beverages work (or don't work) for each condition, you will need to take control of your particular situation to find what works best for you. If your condition persists, seek professional guidance for clarification and a specialized dietary plan.

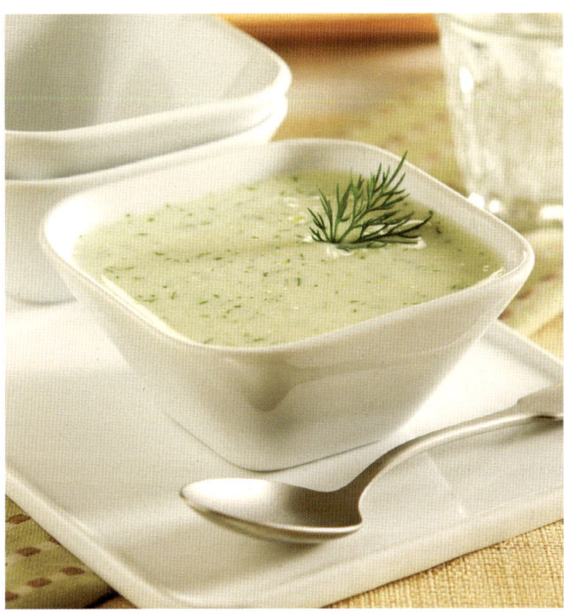

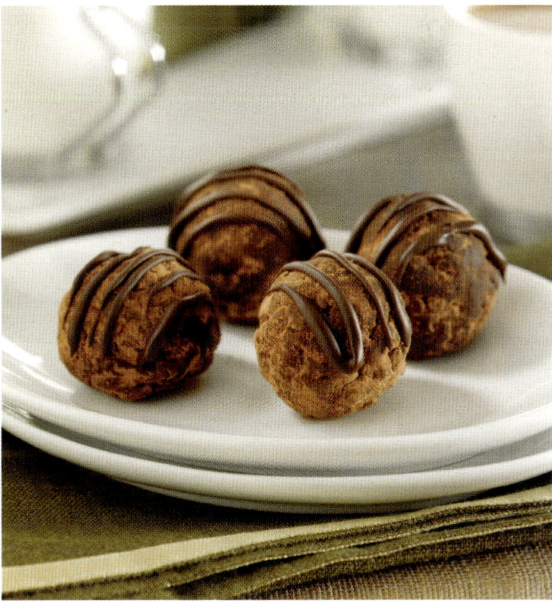

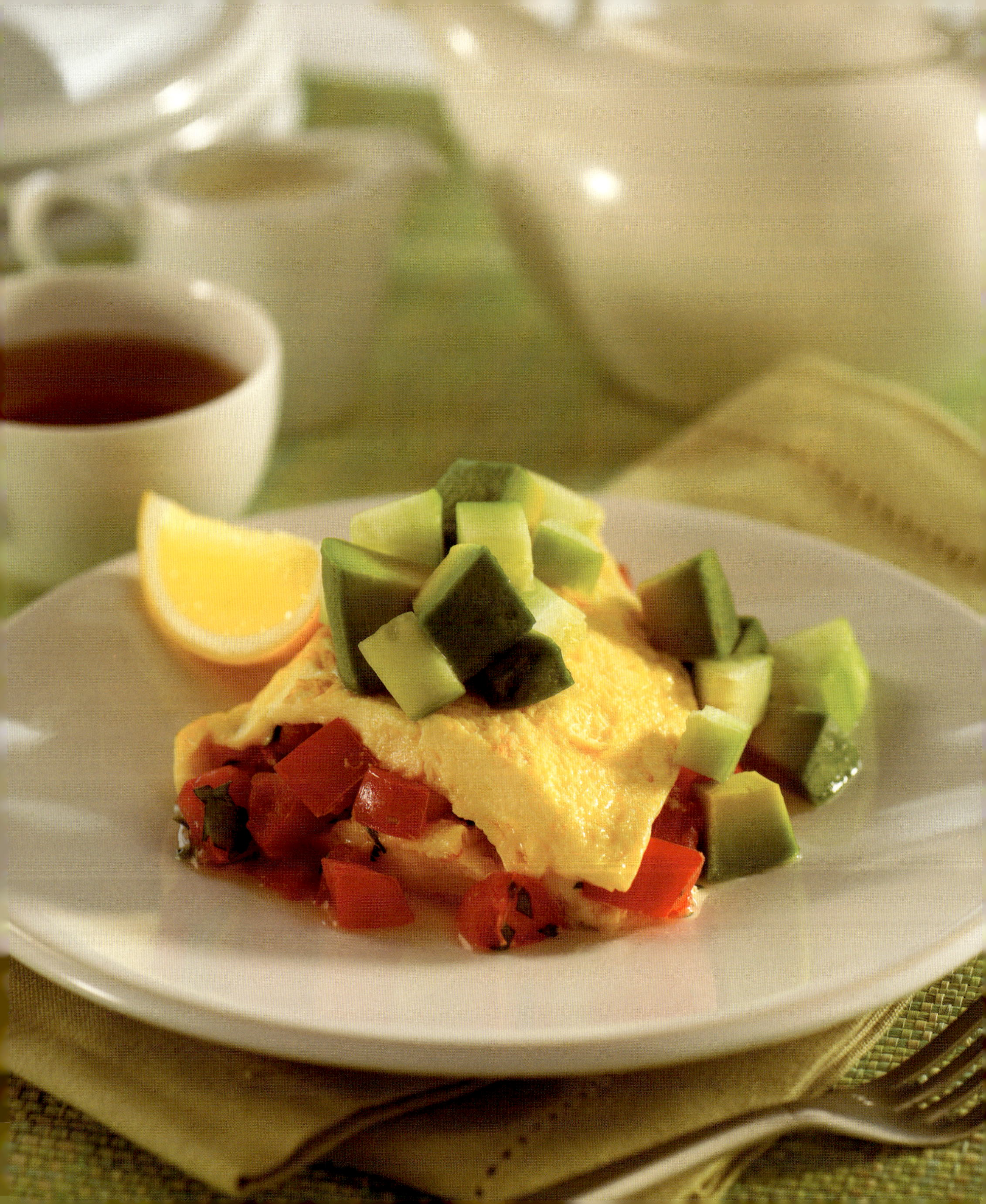

BREAKFAST & BRUNCH

California Omelet with Avocado

makes 2 servings

- **1 plum tomato, chopped**
- **2 to 4 tablespoons chopped fresh cilantro**
- **¼ teaspoon salt**
- **6 eggs**
- **¼ cup almond milk**
- **1 ripe medium avocado, diced**
- **1 small cucumber, chopped**
- **1 lemon, quartered**

1. Preheat oven to 200°F. Combine tomato, cilantro and salt in small bowl; set aside.
2. Whisk eggs and milk in medium bowl until well blended.
3. Heat small nonstick ovenproof skillet over medium heat; spray with nonstick cooking spray. Pour half of egg mixture into skillet; cook 2 minutes or until eggs begin to set. Lift edge of omelet to allow uncooked portion to flow underneath. Cook 3 minutes or until set.
4. Spoon half of tomato mixture over half of omelet. Loosen omelet with spatula and fold in half. Slide omelet onto serving plate and keep warm. Repeat for second omelet. Top with avocado and cucumber. Garnish with lemon.

Super Oatmeal

makes 5 to 6 servings

- 2 cups water
- 2¾ cups old-fashioned oats
- ¼ cup finely diced dried figs
- ¼ cup lightly packed dark brown sugar
- ⅓ to ½ cup sliced almonds, toasted*
- ¼ cup flaxseeds
- ½ teaspoon salt
- ½ teaspoon ground cinnamon
- 2 cups almond milk

**To toast almonds, spread on small baking sheet. Bake in preheated 350°F oven 8 to 10 minutes or until golden brown, stirring frequently.*

1. Bring water to a boil in large saucepan over high heat. Stir in oats, figs, brown sugar, almonds, flaxseeds, salt and cinnamon. Immediately add milk; stir until well blended.
2. Reduce heat to medium-high. Cook and stir 5 to 7 minutes or until oatmeal is thick and creamy. Spoon into individual bowls.

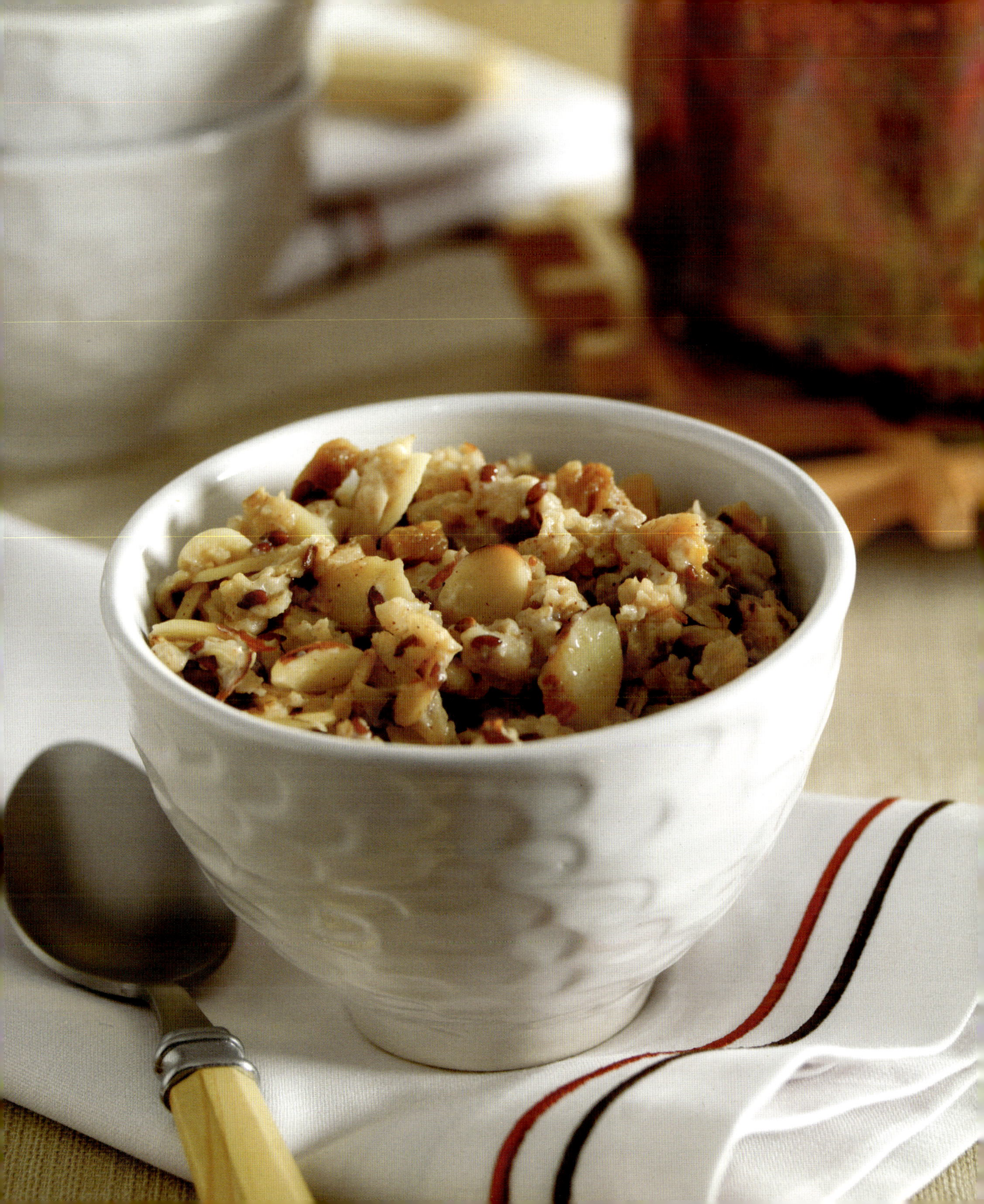

Scrambled Egg and Zucchini Pie

makes 2 servings

2 eggs

1 tablespoon grated Parmesan or Cheddar cheese (optional)

¼ teaspoon salt

1 teaspoon olive oil

1 small zucchini, diced

1. Preheat oven to 350°F.
2. Whisk eggs in small bowl; stir in cheese, if desired, and salt.
3. Heat oil in small ovenproof nonstick skillet over medium-high heat. Add zucchini; cook and stir 2 to 3 minutes or until crisp-tender.
4. Reduce heat to low; stir egg mixture into skillet with zucchini. Cook without stirring 4 to 5 minutes or until eggs begin to set around edge.
5. Transfer skillet to oven and bake 5 minutes or until eggs are set. Cut into wedges to serve.

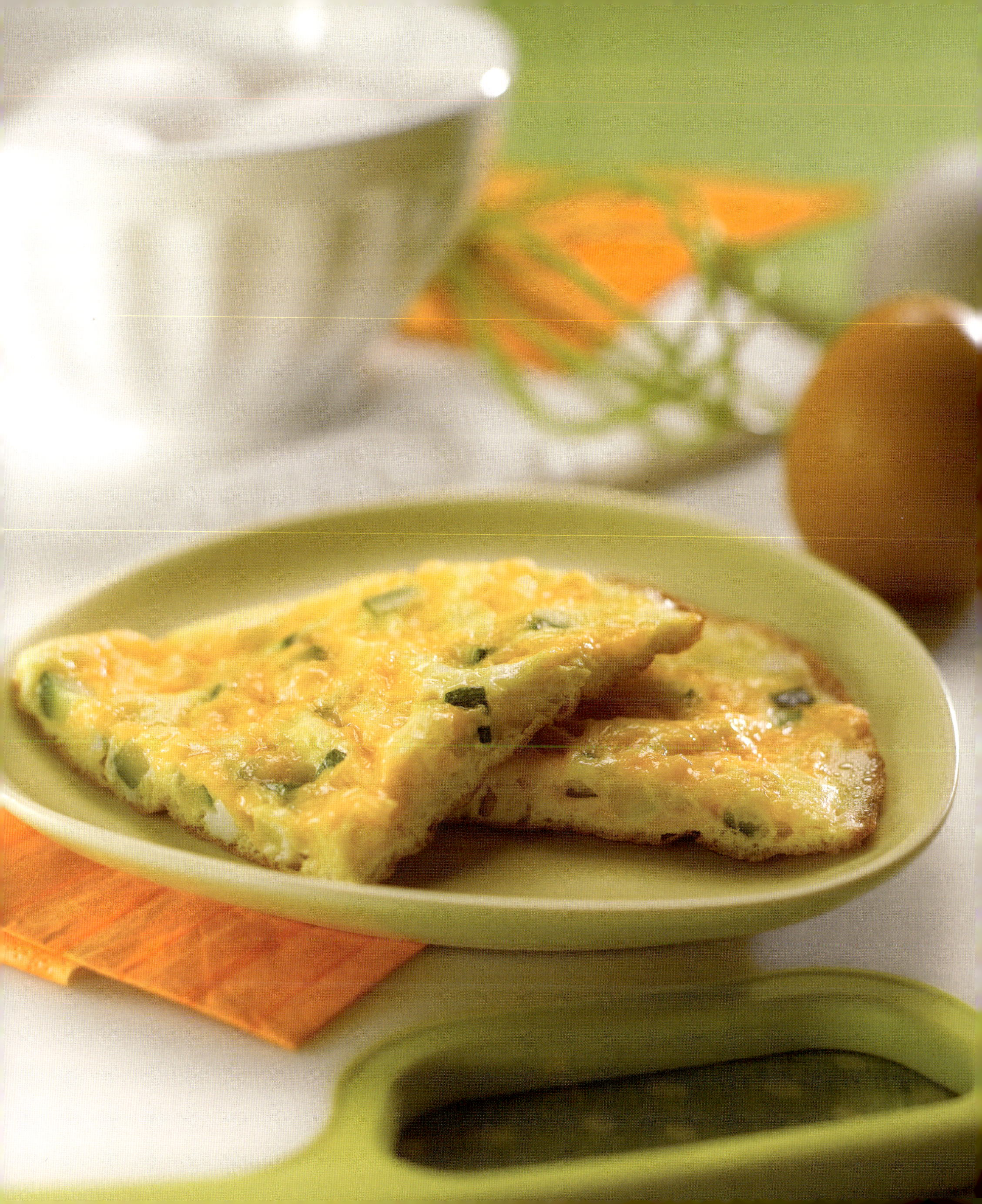

Hash Brown Frittata

makes 2 servings

¾ cup coarsely chopped cherry tomatoes

½ cup refrigerated hash brown potatoes

¼ teaspoon salt, divided (optional)

¼ teaspoon black pepper, divided

4 eggs

⅛ teaspoon red pepper flakes

¼ cup salsa (optional)

1. Preheat broiler. Spray large ovenproof nonstick skillet with nonstick cooking spray. Add tomatoes. Cook over medium heat 5 minutes or until tomatoes are pulpy, stirring frequently. Add potatoes; press into tomato mixture. Cook over medium heat 5 minutes or until potatoes begin to turn golden. Sprinkle with ⅛ teaspoon salt, if desired, and ⅛ teaspoon black pepper.
2. Combine remaining salt, if desired, and black pepper, eggs and red pepper flakes in small bowl. Pour into skillet, coating potato mixture. Cook over medium heat until egg mixture is set, turning skillet as needed to cook egg mixture completely.
3. Place skillet in broiler 4 or 5 inches from heat 30 seconds or until egg is set. Cut frittata into wedges. Serve with salsa, if desired.

NOTE Refrigerated hash brown potatoes are usually available in the produce or egg section of the supermarket.

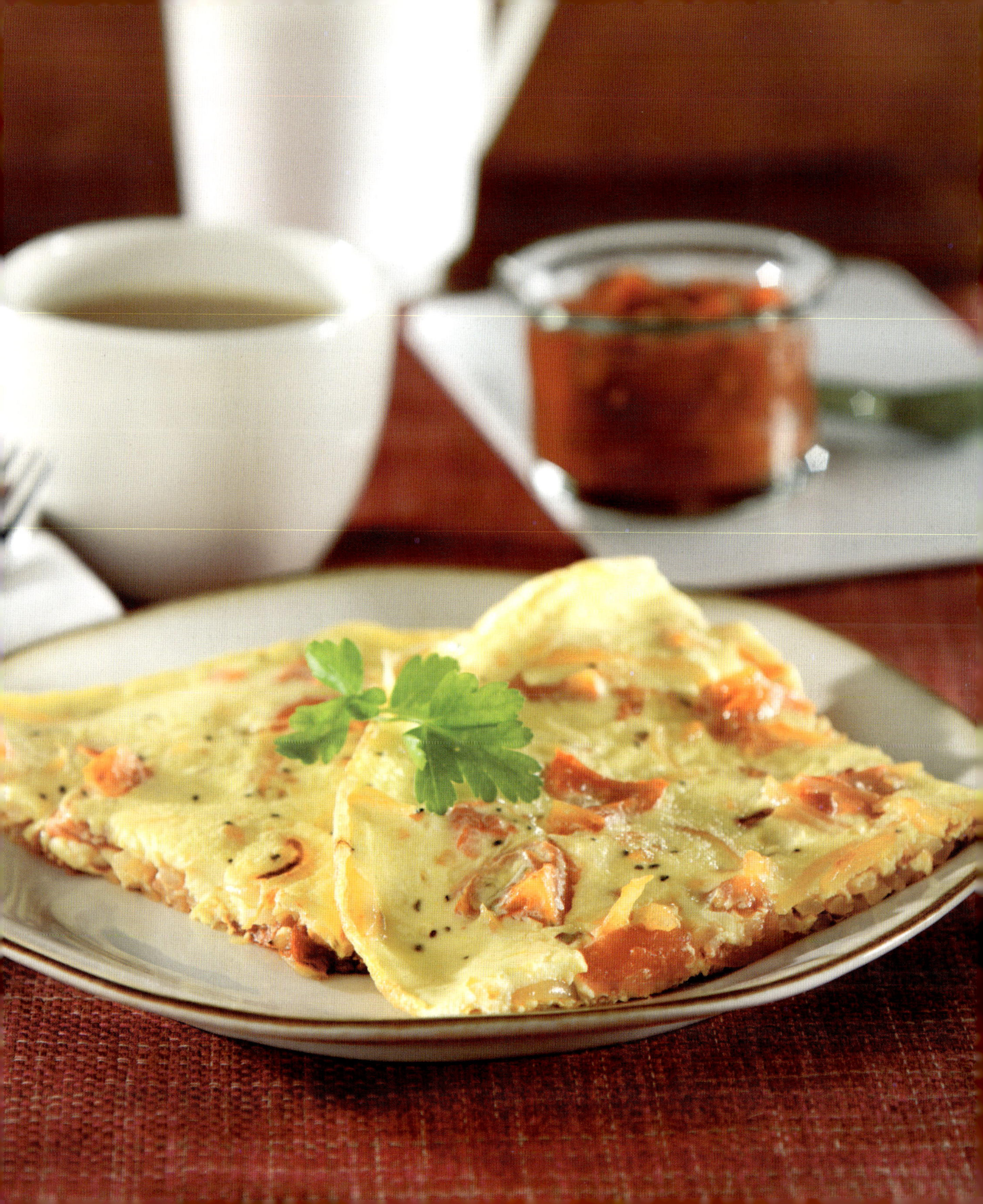

Scrambled Egg Pile Ups

makes 1 serving

- **2 eggs**
- **2 tablespoons almond milk**
- **Salt and black pepper**
- **¼ cup diced orange bell pepper**
- **1 green onion (green part only), finely chopped**
- **¼ cup grape tomatoes, quartered (about 6 tomatoes)**
- **⅓ cup (about 1½ ounces) shredded Cheddar cheese (optional)**

1. Preheat waffle maker to medium; spray with nonstick cooking spray.
2. Whisk eggs and milk in small bowl. Season lightly with salt and black pepper. Working quickly, pour egg mixture onto waffle maker, sprinkle with bell pepper, green onion and tomatoes. Close; cook 2 minutes or until puffed.
3. Remove "waffle" to plate; top with cheese, if desired. Serve immediately.

TIP To remove from the waffle maker, place a plate over the egg and flip the egg onto the plate. Or, use the tip of a fork to gently release the egg from the waffle maker, then slide a wide spatula under the egg to transfer it to a plate.

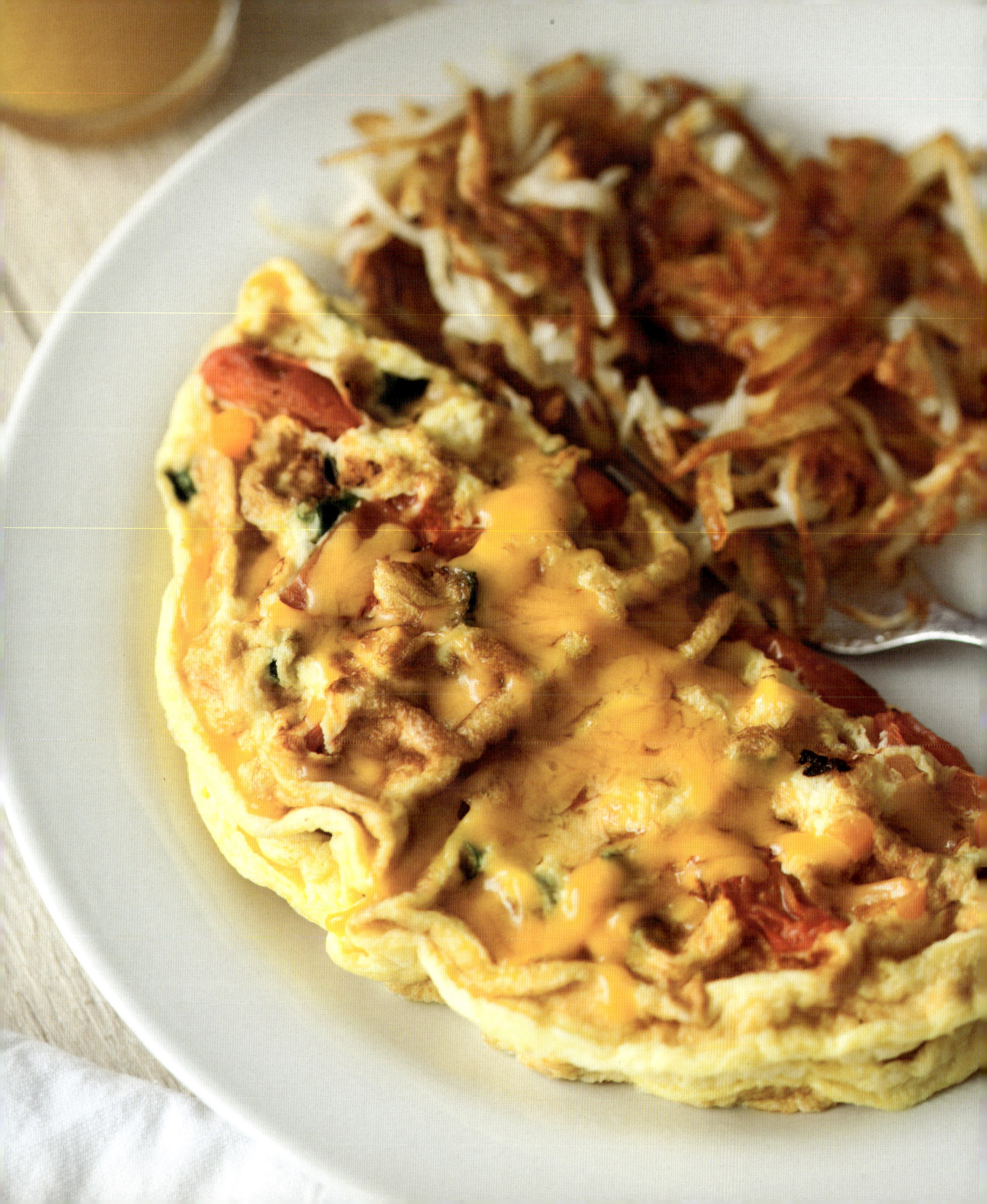

Vegetable Quinoa Frittata

makes 6 servings

- 1 tablespoon olive oil
- 1 cup small broccoli florets
- ¾ cup finely chopped red bell pepper
- ½ teaspoon garlic powder
- 1¼ teaspoons kosher salt
- Black pepper
- 1½ cups cooked quinoa
- ¼ cup sun-dried tomatoes (packed in oil), chopped
- 8 eggs, lightly beaten
- ¼ cup grated Parmesan cheese (optional)

1. Preheat oven to 400°F.
2. Heat oil in large ovenproof nonstick skillet over medium-high heat. Add broccoli; cook and stir 4 minutes, Add bell pepper; cook and stir 2 minutes. Add garlic powder, salt and black pepper; cook 30 seconds, stirring constantly. Stir in quinoa and sun-dried tomatoes.
3. Gently stir in eggs; cook until softly scrambled. Sprinkle with cheese, if desired.
4. Bake about 7 minutes or until eggs are set. Let stand 5 minutes before cutting into wedges.

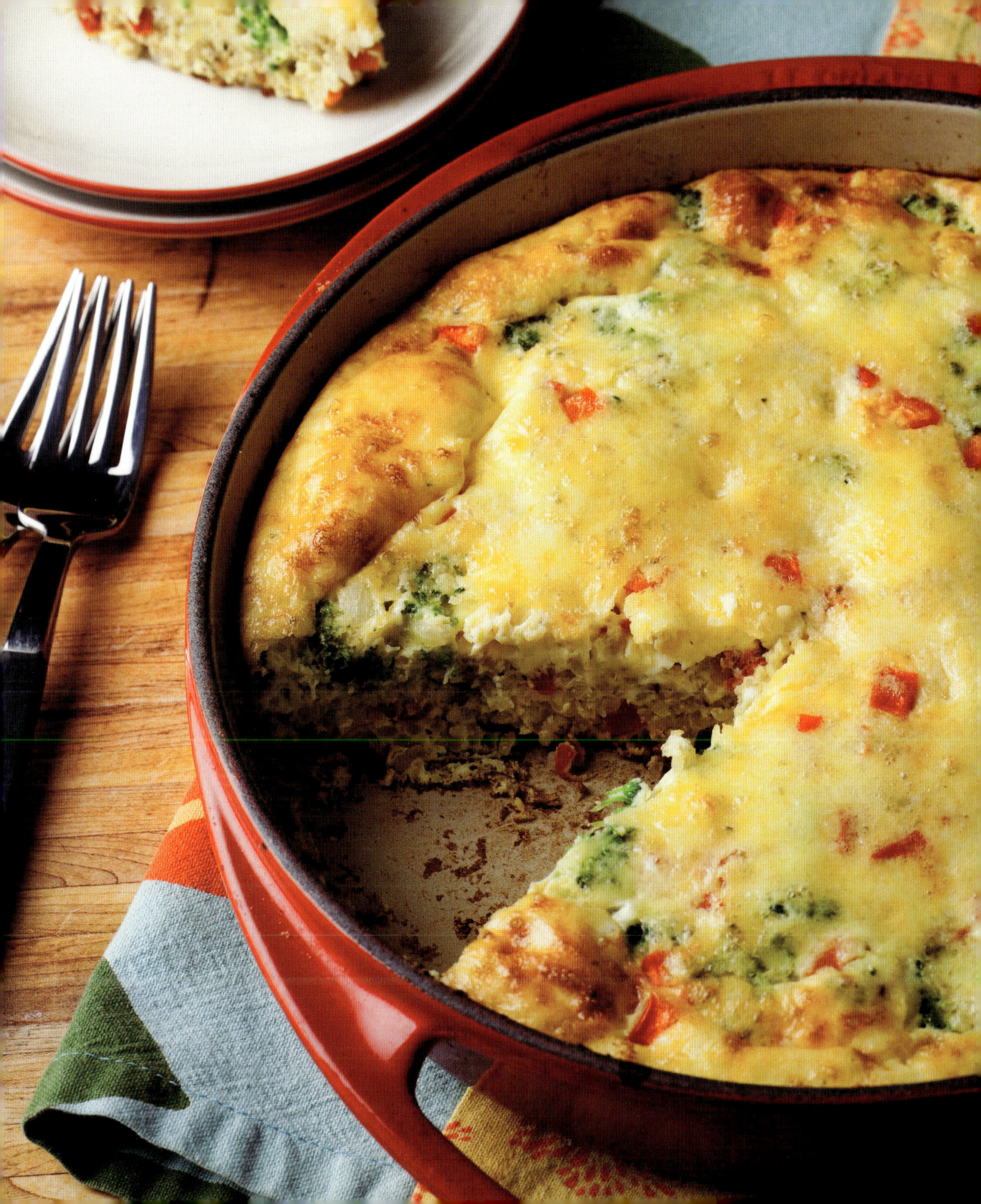

Sizzling Rice Flour Crêpes

makes 4 to 6 servings

Crêpes

1 cup rice flour
½ teaspoon salt
½ teaspoon sugar
½ teaspoon turmeric
1 cup unsweetened coconut milk
½ to ¾ cup water
½ cup vegetable oil

Filling

1 bunch green onions (green parts only), chopped
1 cup chopped cooked chicken *or* 1 cup small raw shrimp, peeled *or* 1 cup cubed tofu
2 cups bean sprouts
Lettuce, fresh cilantro and fresh mint

Dipping Sauce (optional)

⅔ cup water
¼ cup gluten-free fish sauce
1 tablespoon sugar
Juice of 1 lime
1 serrano or other hot pepper, minced
1 to 2 tablespoons shredded carrot

1. Combine rice flour, salt, sugar and turmeric in medium bowl. Gradually whisk in coconut milk and ½ cup water until batter is thickness of heavy cream. Let batter rest at least 10 minutes. Add additional water as needed to thin batter.
2. Heat 9- or 10-inch nonstick skillet over medium heat. Add 3 teaspoons oil to skillet. Add choice of ¼ cup filling to skillet (about 1 tablespoon green onion, plus 3 tablespoons chicken, shrimp, tofu or a combination). Cook and stir 2 to 4 minutes or until onions are softened and shrimp is pink and opaque, if using. Pour about ½ cup batter over filling mixture. Immediately swirl to coat bottom of pan with batter; allow some batter to go up side of pan.
3. In 30 seconds or when sizzling sound stops, add bean sprouts to 1 side of crêpe. Cover pan and cook 3 minutes or until sprouts wilt and center of crêpe appears cooked. Edges should be browned and crisp.
4. Fold crêpe in half with spatula and transfer to plate. Repeat with remaining batter and fillings.
5. For Dipping Sauce, if desired, combine ⅔ cup water, fish sauce, sugar and lime juice in small bowl. Stir until sugar dissolves. Stir in pepper; top with carrot.

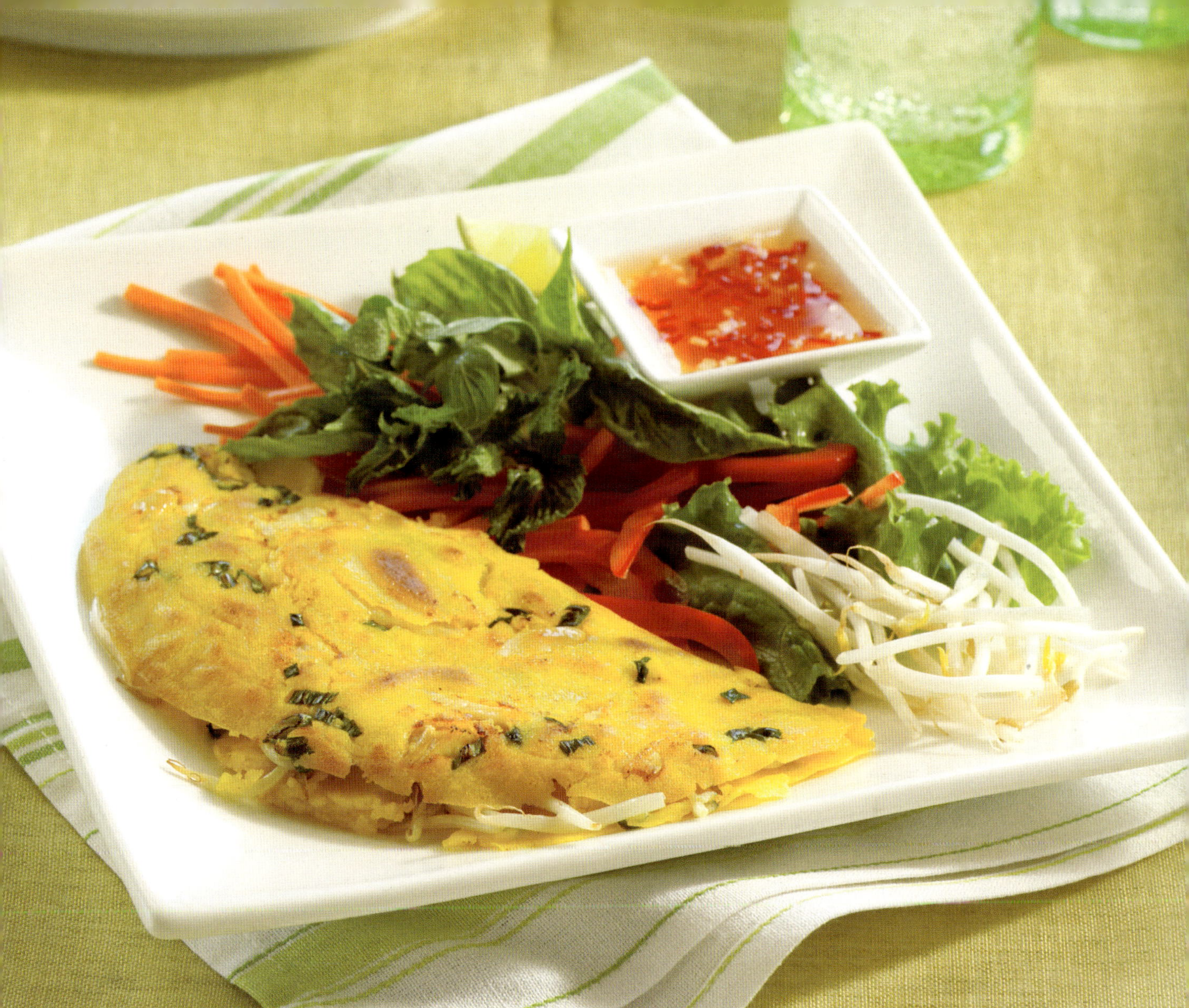

6. Serve crêpes with lettuce, herbs and Dipping Sauce, if desired. Traditionally, crêpes are eaten by wrapping bite-size portions in lettuce with herbs and dipping each bite in sauce.

TIP Sizzling Crêpes (Banh Xeo, pronounced bahn SAY-oh) are a popular Vietnamese street snack. The word "Xeo" in Vietnamese mimics the sound the batter makes as it sizzles in the pan. The filling can be almost anything you wish. Try using leftover pork, beef, vegetables or whatever you have on hand. Part of the experience is choosing which fresh herbs to add to each portion of the crêpe before wrapping it in a lettuce leaf and dipping it in sauce. Banh Xeo are a truly hands-on eating experience!

Superfood Breakfast Porridge

makes 4 servings

- ¾ cup steel-cut oats
- ¼ cup uncooked quinoa, rinsed and drained
- 2 tablespoons dried cranberries
- 2 tablespoons raisins
- 3 tablespoons ground flaxseeds
- 2 tablespoons chia seeds
- 1 teaspoon olive oil
- ¼ teaspoon salt
- ¼ teaspoon ground cinnamon
- 2½ cups almond milk, plus additional for serving
- 1½ cups water
- Maple syrup (optional)
- ¼ cup sliced almonds, toasted* (optional)

****To toast almonds, cook and stir in small skillet over medium heat 1 to 2 minutes or until lightly browned.***

Slow Cooker Directions

1. Combine oats, quinoa, cranberries, raisins, flaxseeds, chia seeds, oil, salt and cinnamon in heatproof bowl that fits inside a slow cooker. Stir in 2½ cups milk until blended.
2. Place bowl in slow cooker. Pour enough water around sides to come up halfway around bowl.
3. Cover; cook on LOW 8 hours.
4. Carefully remove bowl from slow cooker. Stir in additional milk. Top with maple syrup and almonds, if desired.

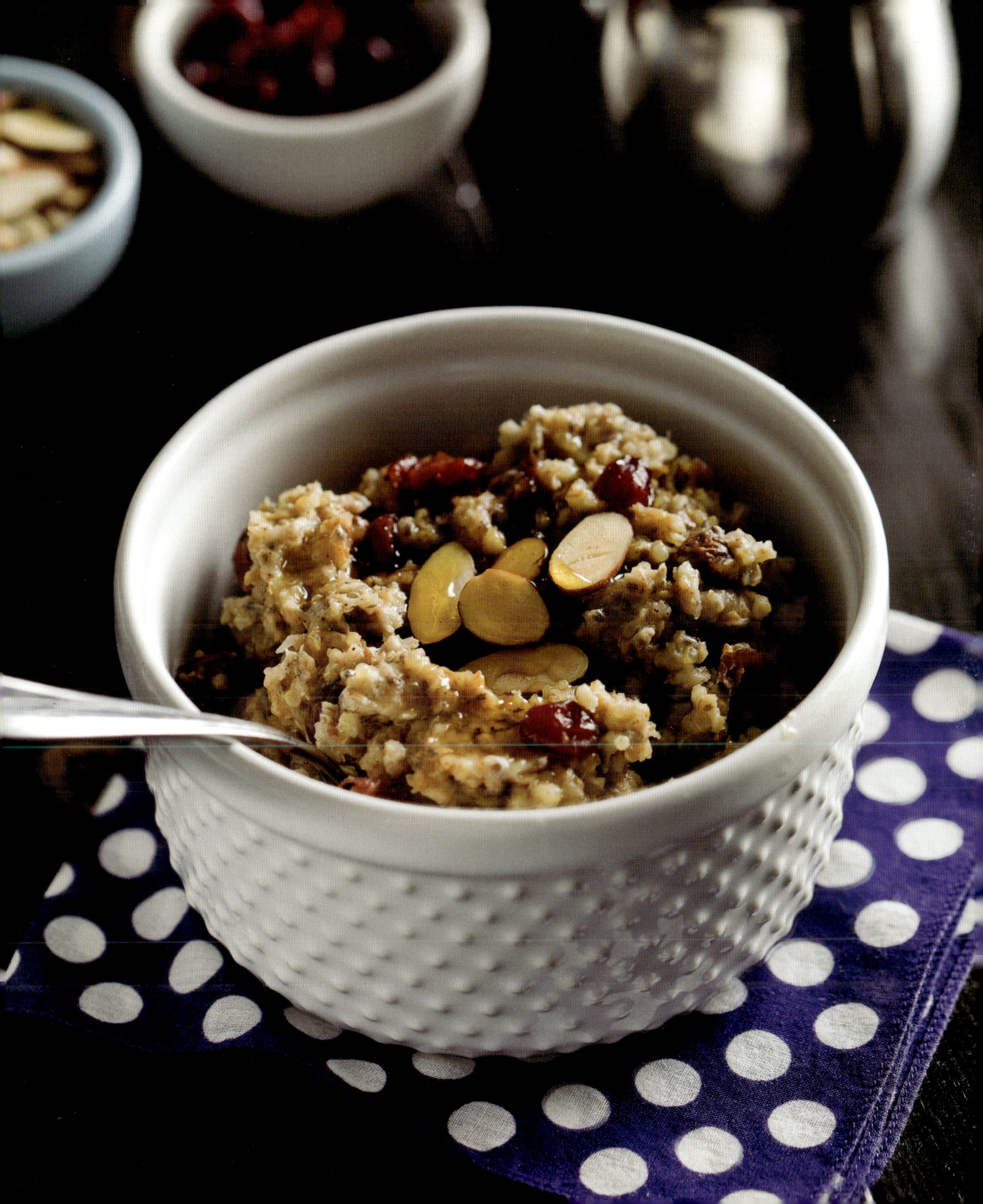

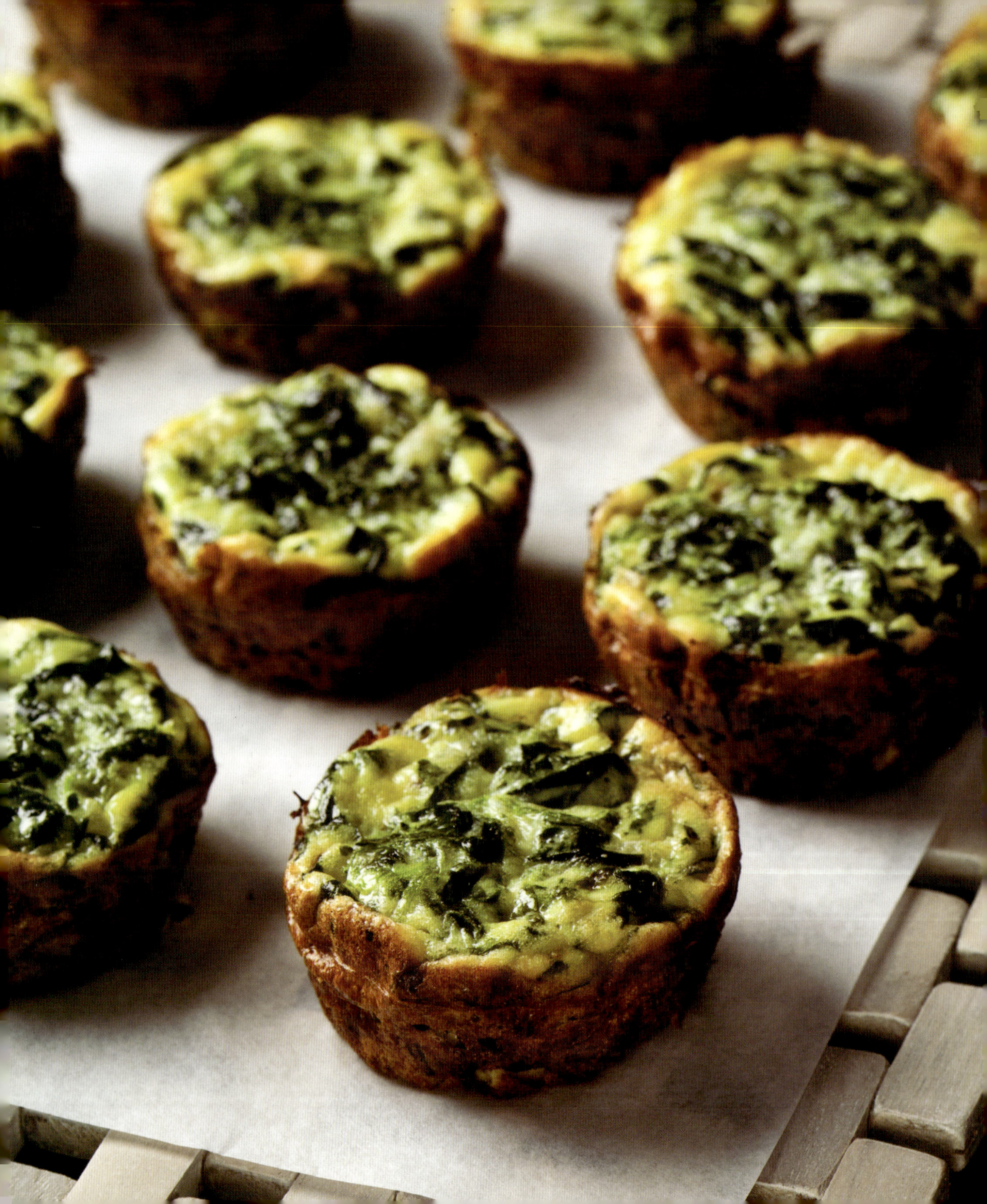

STARTERS & APPETIZERS

Mini Spinach Frittatas

makes 12 mini frittatas (4 to 6 servings)

8 eggs
¼ cup plain nonfat Greek yogurt
1 package (10 ounces) frozen chopped spinach, thawed and squeezed dry
¼ cup (2 ounces) shredded white Cheddar cheese
¼ cup grated Parmesan cheese
¾ teaspoon salt
⅛ teaspoon black pepper
⅛ teaspoon ground red pepper
Dash ground nutmeg
1 tablespoon olive oil

1. Preheat oven to 350°F. Spray 12 standard (2½-inch) muffin cups with nonstick cooking spray.
2. Whisk eggs and yogurt in large bowl. Stir in spinach, Cheddar and Parmesan cheeses, salt, black pepper, red pepper and nutmeg until blended. Divide mixture evenly among prepared muffin cups.
3. Bake 20 to 25 minutes or until eggs are puffed and firm and no longer shiny. Cool in pan 2 minutes. Loosen bottom and sides with small spatula or knife; remove to wire rack. Serve warm, cold or at room temperature.

Vegetable-Topped Hummus

makes 8 servings

- 1 can (about 15 ounces) chickpeas, rinsed and drained
- 2 tablespoons tahini
- 2 tablespoons lemon juice
- ½ teaspoon garlic powder
- ¾ teaspoon salt
- 1 tomato, finely chopped
- 2 green onions, finely chopped
- 2 tablespoons chopped fresh parsley
- Oat crackers or fresh vegetable slices (optional)

1. Combine chickpeas, tahini, lemon juice, garlic powder and salt in food processor or blender; process until smooth.
2. Combine tomato, green onions and parsley in small bowl; gently toss to combine.
3. Spoon hummus into serving bowl; top with tomato mixture. Serve with crackers or vegetable slices, if desired.

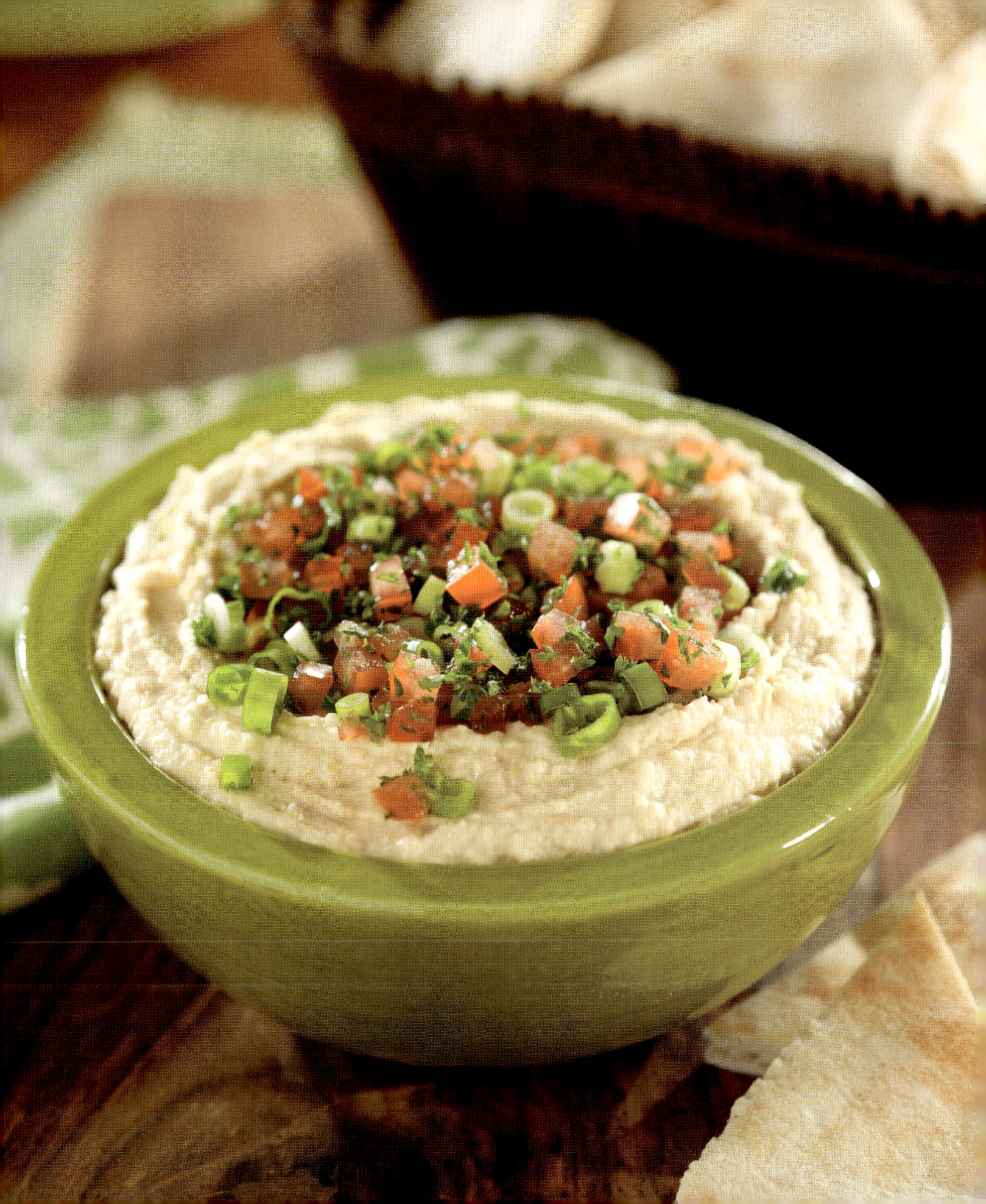

Guacamole

makes 2 cups

- 2 large ripe avocados
- 2 teaspoons fresh lime juice
- ¼ cup finely chopped red onion (optional)
- 2 tablespoons chopped fresh cilantro
- ½ jalapeño pepper,* finely chopped
- ½ teaspoon salt

***Jalapeño peppers can sting and irritate the skin, so wear rubber gloves when handling peppers and do not touch your eyes.**

1. Place avocados in large bowl. Sprinkle with lime juice; toss to coat. Mash to desired consistency with fork or potato masher.
2. Add onion, if desired, cilantro, jalapeño pepper and salt; stir gently until well blended.

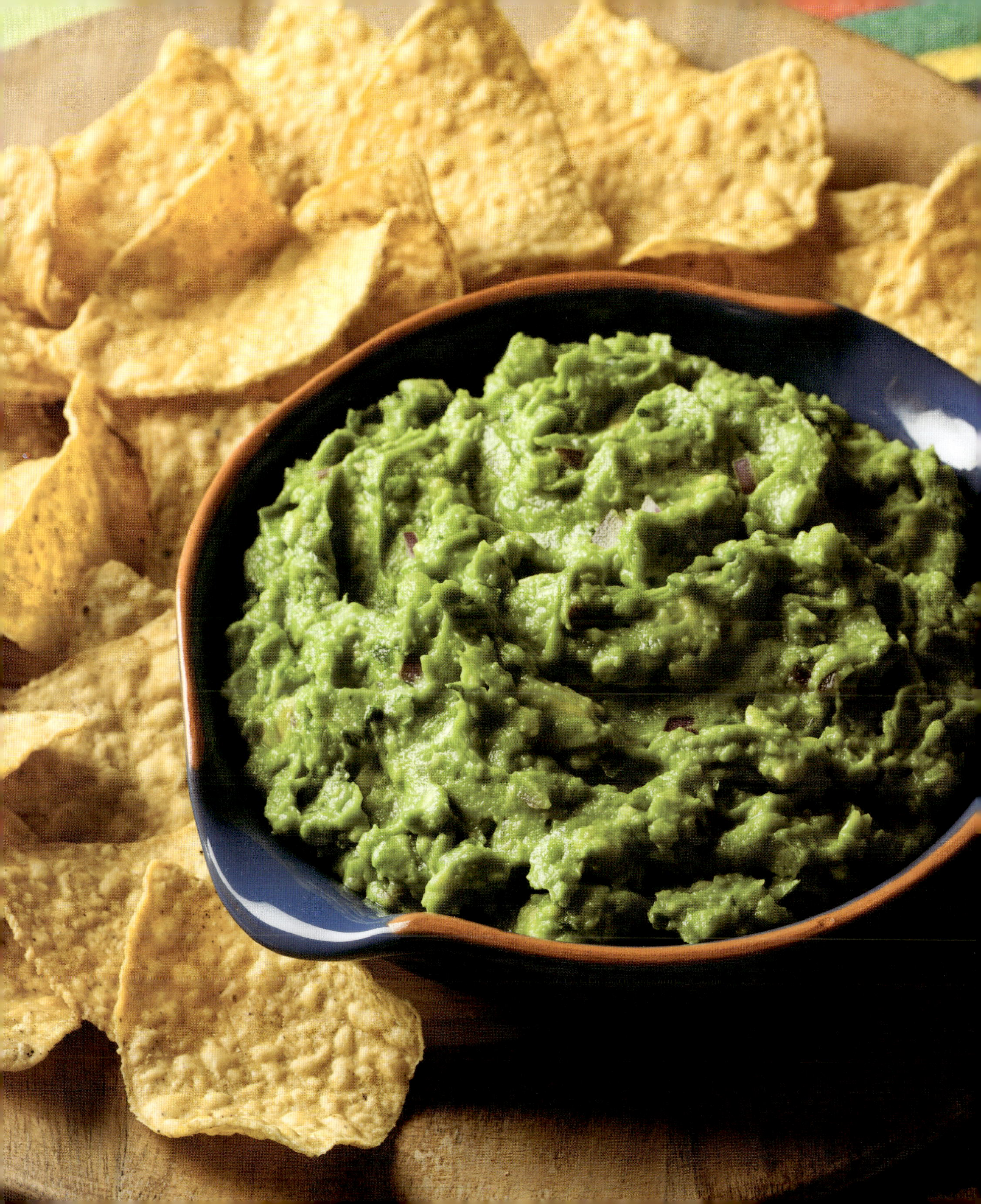

Thai Coconut Chicken Meatballs

makes 4 to 5 servings

- **1 pound ground chicken**
- **2 green onions, chopped**
- **½ teaspoon garlic powder**
- **2 teaspoons dark sesame oil**
- **2 teaspoons mirin**
- **1 teaspoon fish sauce**
- **1 tablespoon canola oil**
- **½ cup unsweetened canned coconut milk**
- **¼ cup chicken broth**
- **1 teaspoon packed brown sugar**
- **1 teaspoon Thai red curry paste**
- **2 teaspoons lime juice**
- **2 tablespoons water**
- **1 tablespoon cornstarch**

Slow Cooker Directions

1. Combine chicken, green onions, garlic powder, sesame oil, mirin and fish sauce in large bowl. Shape mixture into 1½-inch meatballs.
2. Heat canola oil in large skillet over medium-high heat. Working in batches, brown meatballs on all sides. Transfer to 4½-quart slow cooker. Add coconut milk, broth, brown sugar and curry paste. Cover; cook on HIGH 3½ to 4 hours. Stir in lime juice.
3. Stir water into cornstarch in small bowl until smooth. Whisk into sauce in slow cooker. Cook, uncovered, on HIGH 10 to 15 minutes or until sauce is slightly thickened.

TIP To ensure your meatballs are the same size, pat the seasoned ground meat into a rectangle, then cut the rectangle into small, equal-size squares. Roll each portion into a smooth ball.

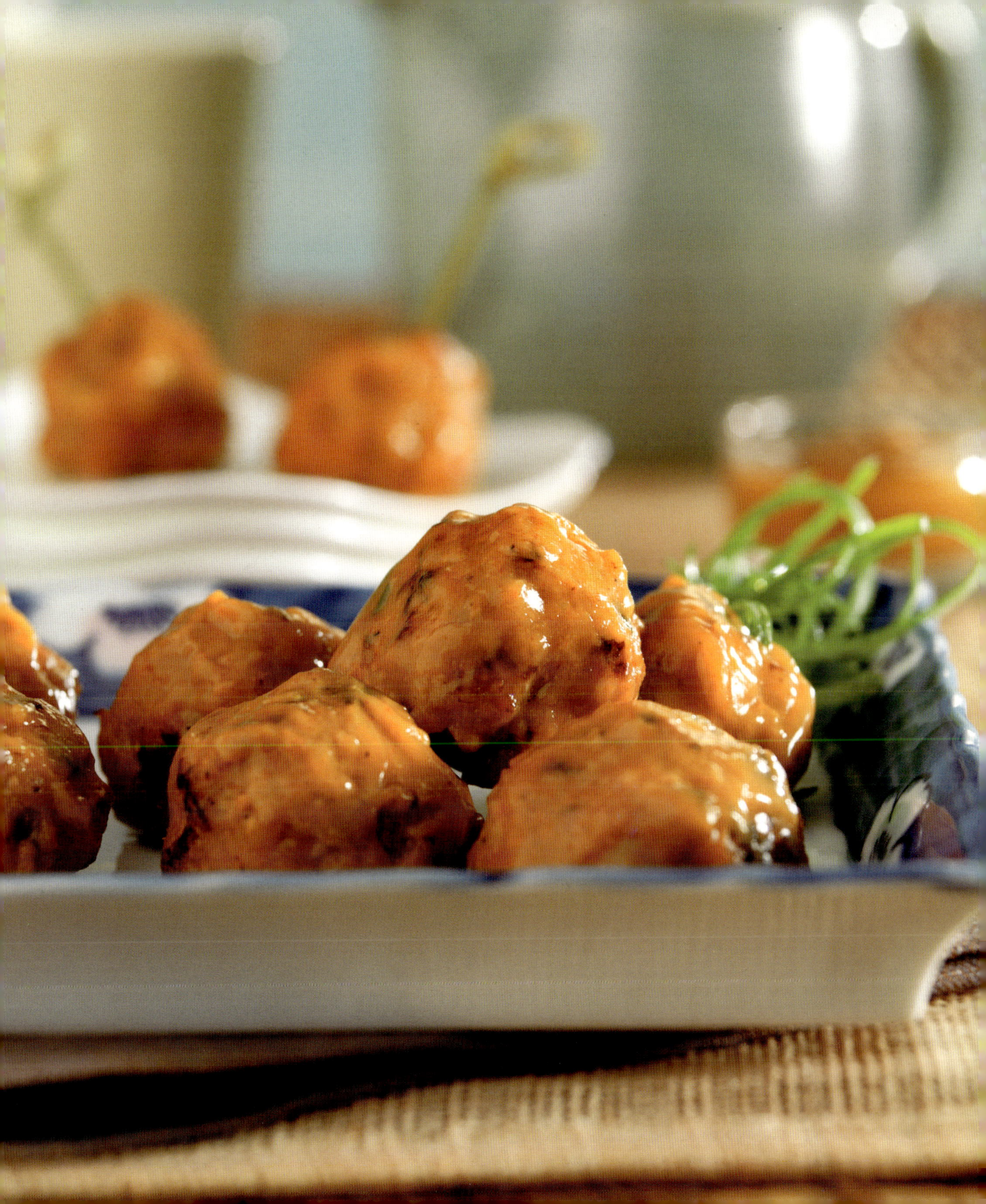

Quick and Easy Hummus

makes 4 servings

- 1 can (about 15 ounces) chickpeas, rinsed and drained
- 2 tablespoons torn fresh mint leaves (optional)
- 2 tablespoons olive oil
- 2 tablespoons lemon juice
- 2 teaspoons dark sesame oil
- ½ teaspoon garlic powder
- ½ teaspoon salt
- ⅛ teaspoon ground red pepper *or* ¼ teaspoon hot pepper sauce

1. With motor running, drop garlic clove through feed tube of food processor; process until finely chopped.
2. Add chickpeas, olive oil, lemon juice, sesame oil, salt and red pepper, if desired; process until well blended and desired consistency is reached. (Process several minutes for very smooth and fluffy hummus.)

SERVING SUGGESTION Serve with vegetable dippers.

TIP Leftover hummus may be covered and refrigerated up to 1 week.

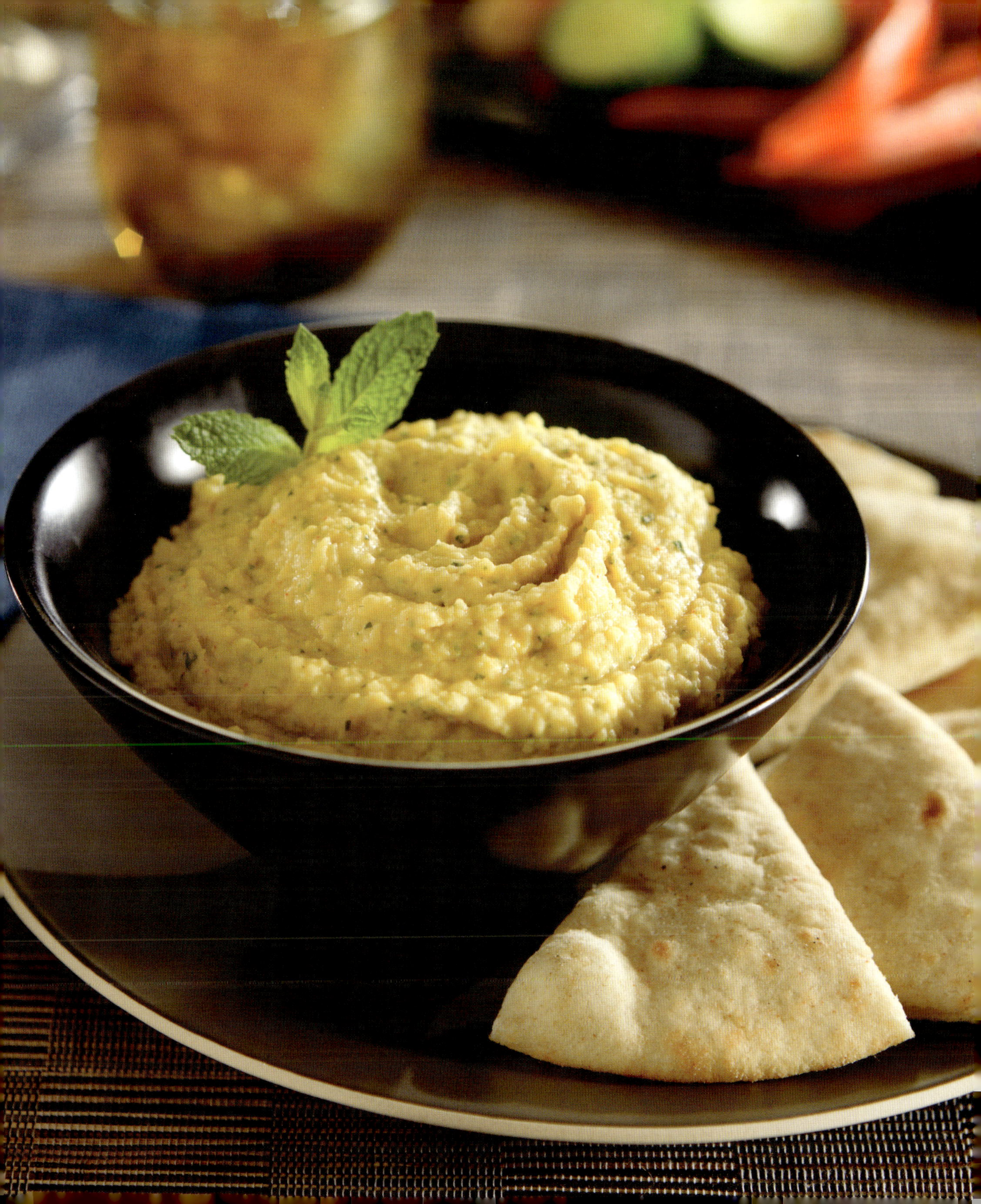

Avocado Smash

makes ¾ cup

- **1 ripe medium avocado**
- **1 tablespoon lime juice**
- **¼ cup plain nonfat Greek yogurt**
- **1 teaspoon Dijon mustard**
- **¼ teaspoon salt**
- **Chopped fresh chives (optional)**

1. Mash avocado in shallow bowl with fork or potato masher until almost smooth.
2. Stir in lime juice, yogurt, mustard and salt until well blended. Sprinkle with chives, if desired. Serve immediately.

TIP This dip is great with raw veggies, such as cucumber slices, celery sticks or red bell pepper strips.

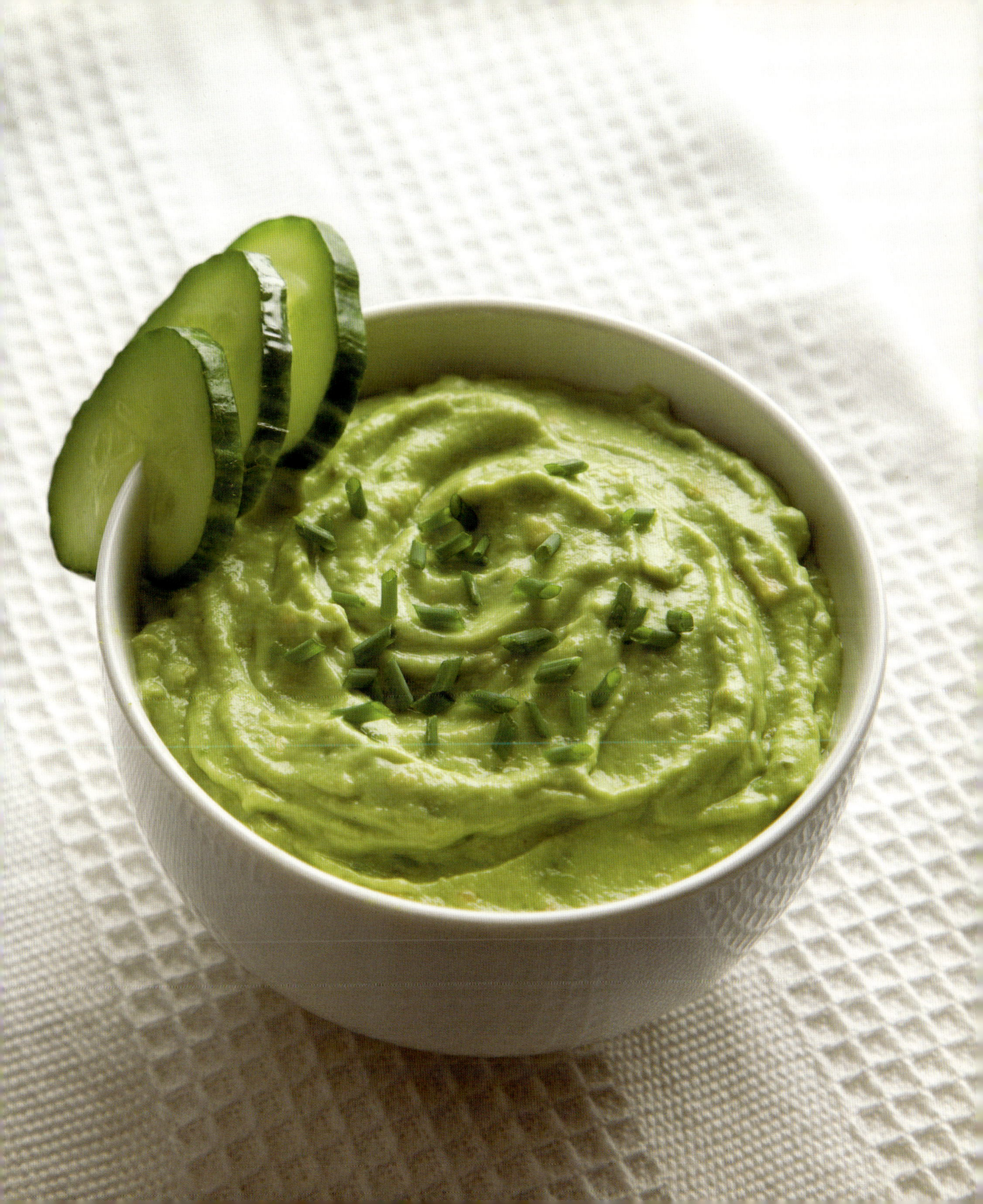

Beef and Lettuce Bundles

makes 8 appetizer servings

- **1 pound ground beef**
- **½ cup green onions, finely chopped**
- **⅔ cup chopped water chestnuts**
- **½ cup chopped red bell pepper**
- **1 tablespoon soy sauce**
- **1 tablespoon seasoned rice vinegar**
- **2 tablespoons chopped fresh cilantro**
- **½ teaspoon garlic powder**
- **1 or 2 heads leaf lettuce, separated into leaves (discard outer leaves)**

1. Brown beef in large skillet over medium-high heat 6 to 8 minutes, stirring to break up meat. Drain fat.
2. Add green onions; cook and stir until tender. Stir in water chestnuts, bell pepper, soy sauce and vinegar; cook until bell pepper is crisp-tender and most of liquid has evaporated, stirring occasionally.
3. Stir in cilantro and garlic powder. Spoon ground beef mixture onto lettuce leaves. Wrap lettuce leaves around beef mixture to make bundles.

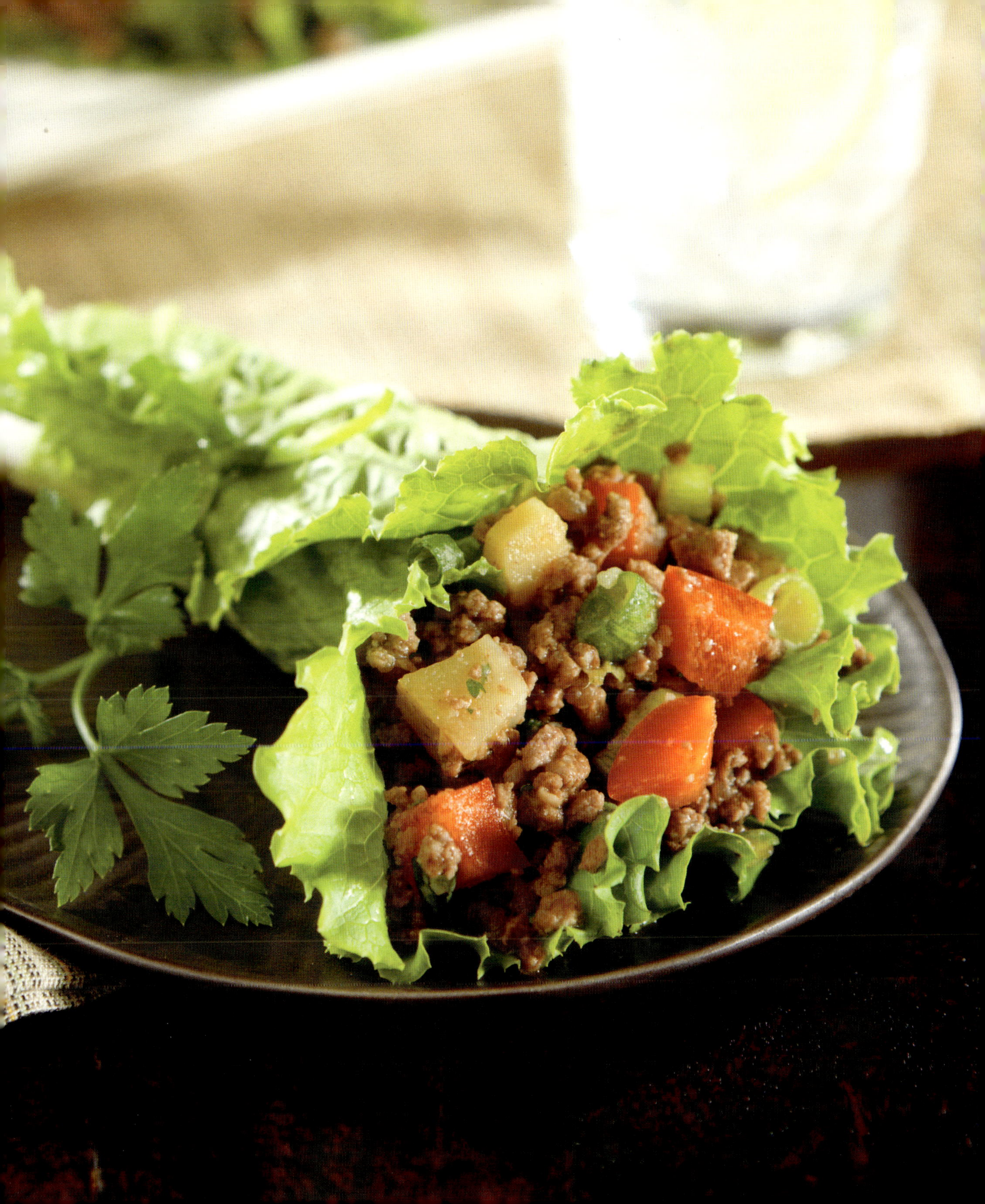

Roasted Eggplant Hummus

makes 2 cups (about 16 servings)

- 1 large eggplant
- 1 can (about 15 ounces) chickpeas, rinsed and drained
- ½ teaspoon garlic powder
- 3 tablespoons fresh lemon juice
- 2 tablespoons olive oil
- ¾ teaspoon salt
- ¼ teaspoon ground red pepper
- ¼ cup loosely packed fresh parsley, plus additional for garnish
- Assorted vegetable sticks and/or gluten-free crackers

1. Preheat oven to 400°F. Cut eggplant in half lengthwise; place cut sides down on baking sheet.
2. Roast 35 to 40 minutes or until tender. Cool completely. Peel eggplant and remove seeds. Reserve pulp.
3. Combine chickpeas and garlic powder food processor; process until finely ground. Add eggplant, lemon juice, oil, salt and ground red pepper; process until smooth. Add ¼ cup parsley; pulse until combined.
4. Serve with assorted vegetables and/or crackers. Garnish with additional parsley.

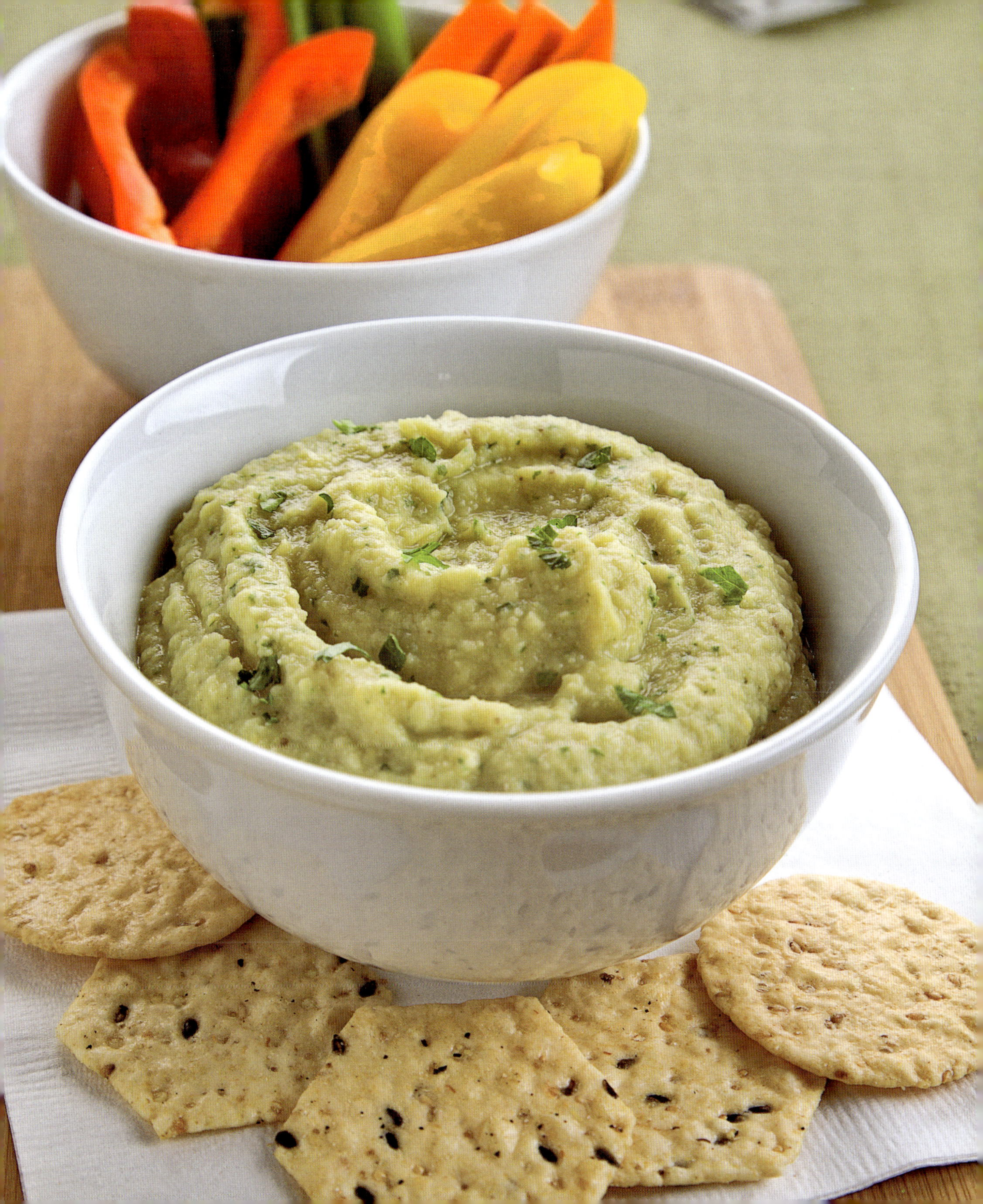

Broiled Shrimp Kabobs

mkes 4 servings

- **2 tablespoons olive oil**
- **2 tablespoons lemon juice**
- **½ teaspoon garlic powder**
- **½ teaspoon salt**
- **½ teaspoon dried oregano**
- **⅛ teaspoon ground red pepper**
- **½ pound medium shrimp, peeled**
- **1 red bell pepper, cut into squares**
- **1 medium zucchini, cut into ½-inch slices**

1. Preheat broiler. Whisk oil, lemon juice, garlic powder, salt, oregano and ground red pepper in medium bowl until well blended. Add shrimp, bell pepper and zucchini; stir to coat.
2. Alternately thread shrimp, bell pepper and zucchini onto skewers.* Place on rack of broiler pan.
3. Broil kabobs 4 inches from heat 2 minutes per side or until shrimp turn pink and opaque.

**If using wooden skewers, soak in water 20 to 30 minutes before threading.*

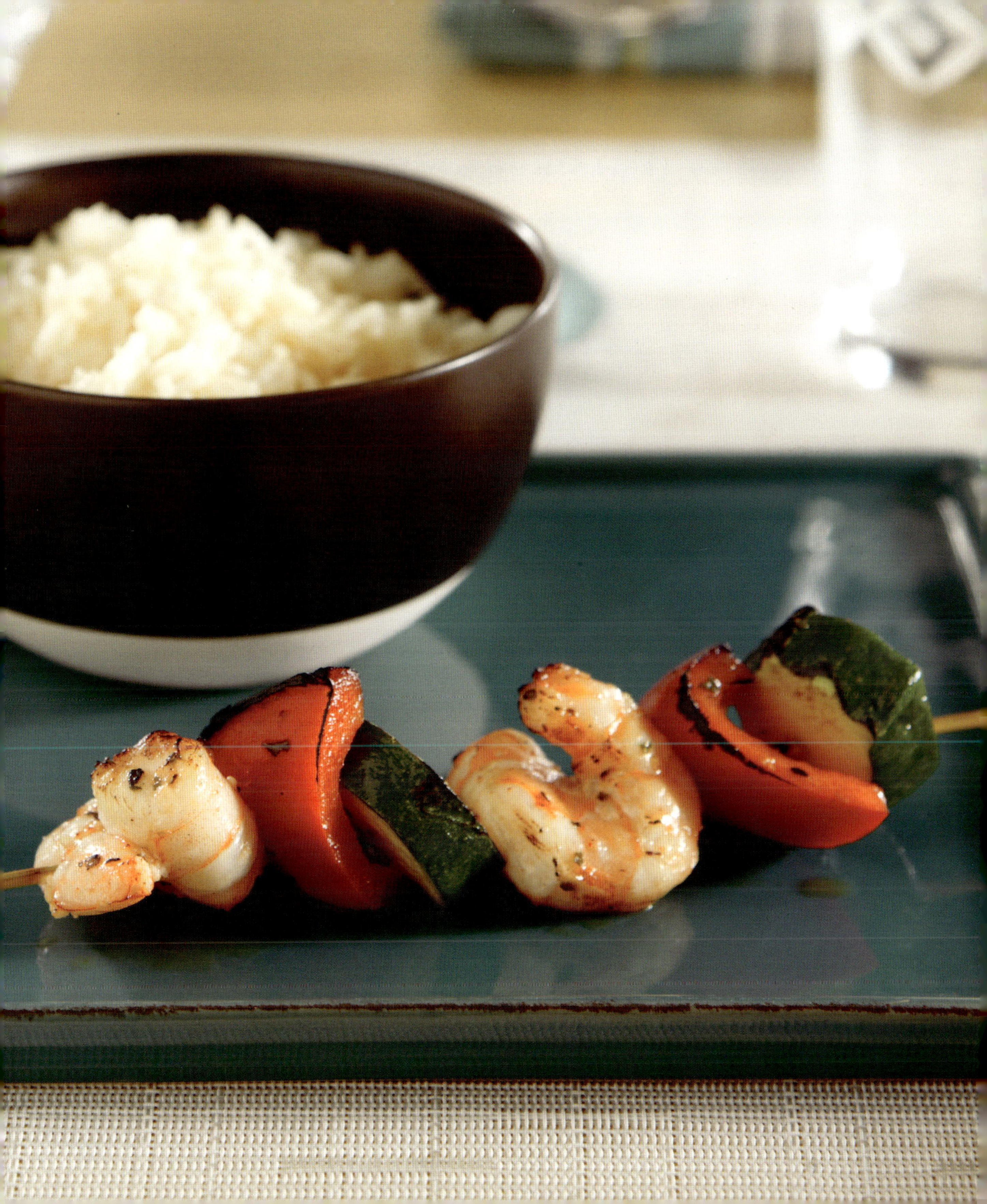

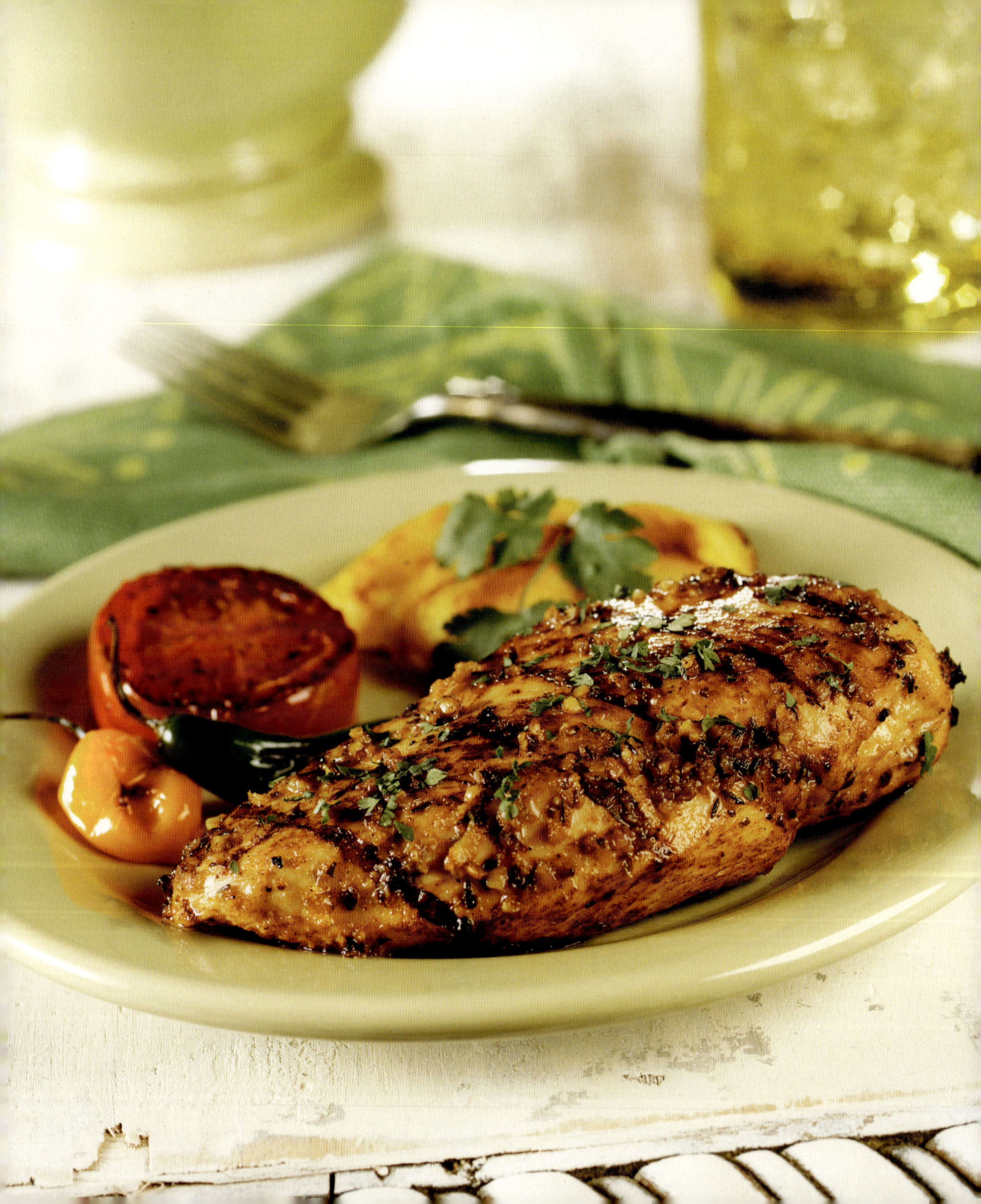

LUNCHES & DINNERS

Grilled Chicken Adobo

makes 6 servings

- ¼ teaspoon onion powder
- ⅓ cup lime juice
- 1 clove garlic, coarsely chopped
- 1 teaspoon ground cumin
- 1 teaspoon dried oregano
- ½ teaspoon dried thyme
- ¼ teaspoon ground red pepper
- 6 boneless skinless chicken breasts (about ¼ pound each)
- 3 tablespoons chopped fresh cilantro (optional)

1. Combine onion powder, lime juice and garlic in large resealable food storage bag. Add cumin, oregano, thyme and ground red pepper; knead bag until blended. Place chicken in bag; press out air and seal. Turn to coat chicken with marinade. Refrigerate 30 minutes or up to 4 hours, turning occasionally.
2. Spray grill grid with nonstick cooking spray. Prepare grill for direct cooking. Remove chicken from marinade; discard marinade.
3. Place chicken on grid. Grill over medium heat 5 to 7 minutes on each side or until chicken is no longer pink in center. Transfer to clean serving platter and garnish with cilantro, if desired.

Lamb Chops with Mustard Sauce

makes 4 servings

- 1 teaspoon dried thyme
- ½ teaspoon salt
- ¼ teaspoon black pepper
- 4 lamb loin chops (about 6 ounces each)
- 2 tablespoons canola or vegetable oil
- 2 tablespoons finely chopped shallots or sweet onion
- ¼ cup beef or chicken broth
- 2 tablespoons Worcestershire sauce
- 1½ tablespoons Dijon mustard
- Sprigs fresh thyme (optional)

1. Sprinkle dried thyme, salt and pepper over lamb. Heat oil in large skillet over medium heat. Add lamb chops; cook 4 minutes per side. Remove to plate; set aside.
2. Add shallots to skillet; cook 3 minutes, stirring occasionally. Reduce heat to medium-low. Add broth, Worcestershire sauce and mustard; simmer 5 minutes or until sauce thickens slightly, stirring occasionally.
3. Return lamb chops to skillet; cook 2 minutes for medium rare, turning once. Transfer to serving plates; garnish with fresh thyme.

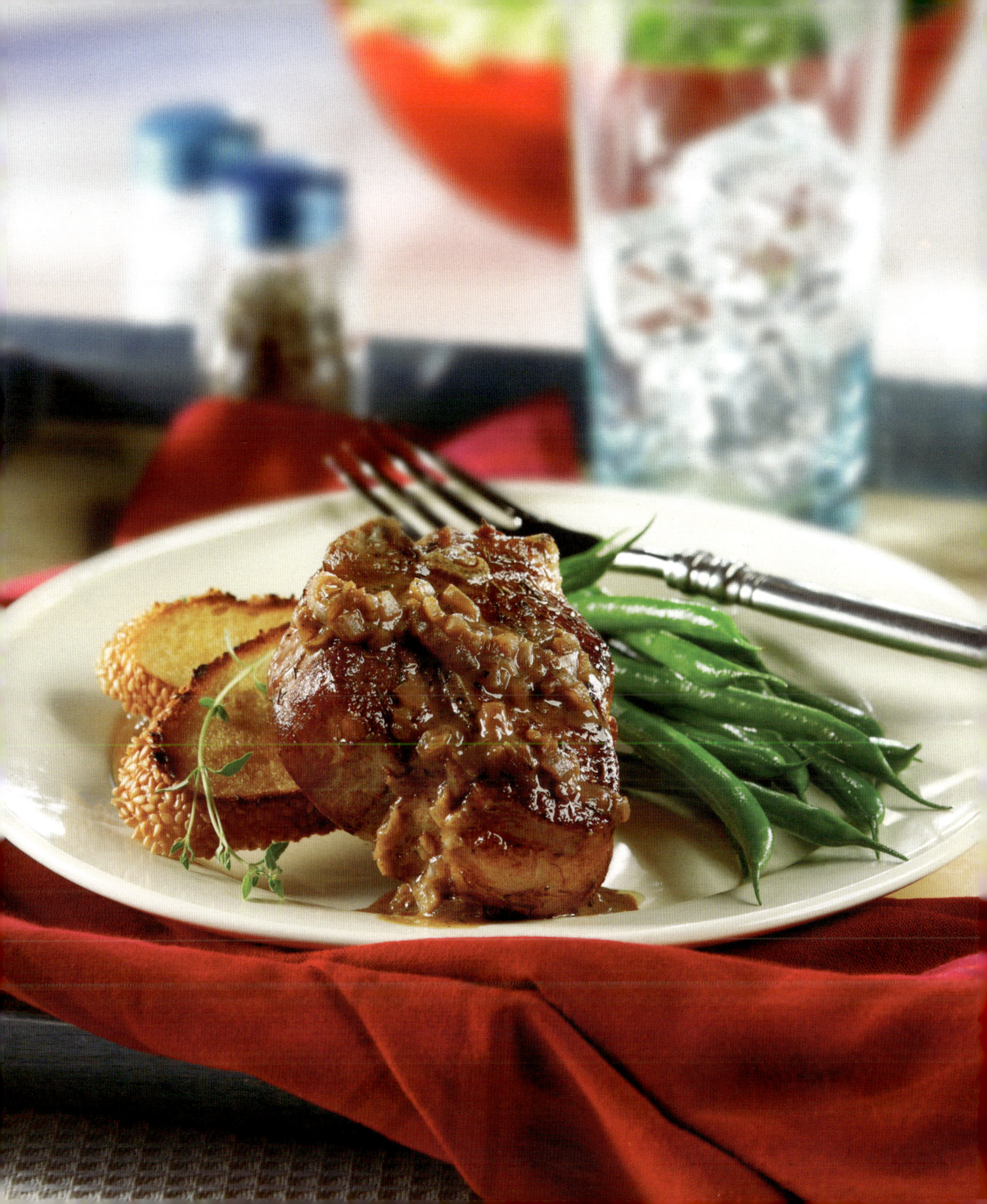

Szechuan Tuna Steaks

makes 4 servings

- **4 tuna steaks (6 ounces each), cut 1 inch thick**
- **¼ cup dry sherry or sake**
- **¼ cup soy sauce**
- **1 tablespoon dark sesame oil**
- **1 teaspoon hot chili oil *or* ¼ teaspoon red pepper flakes**
- **½ teaspoon garlic powder**
- **3 tablespoons chopped fresh cilantro (optional)**

1. Place tuna in single layer in large shallow glass dish. Combine sherry, soy sauce, sesame oil, hot chili oil and garlic powder in small bowl. Reserve ¼ cup soy sauce mixture at room temperature. Pour remaining soy sauce mixture over tuna. Cover and marinate in refrigerator 40 minutes, turning once.
2. Spray grill grid with nonstick cooking spray. Prepare grill for direct cooking. Drain tuna, discarding marinade.
3. Grill tuna, uncovered, over medium-high heat 6 minutes or until tuna is seared but still feels somewhat soft in center,* turning halfway through grilling time. Transfer tuna to cutting board. Cut each tuna steak into thin slices; fan out slices onto serving plates. Drizzle tuna with reserved soy sauce mixture; garnish with cilantro.

**Tuna becomes dry and tough if overcooked. Cook to medium doneness for best results.*

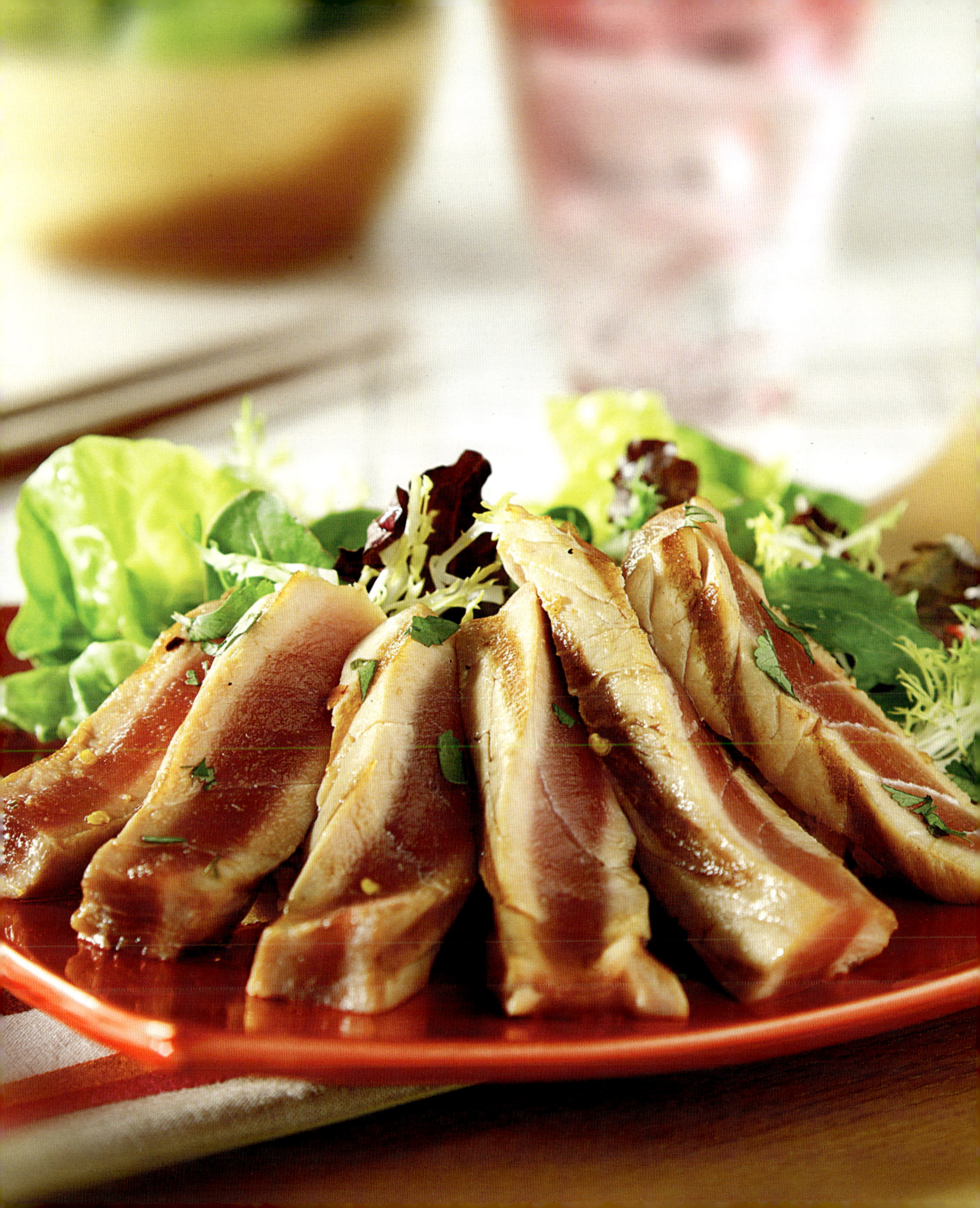

Speedy Salmon Patties

makes 3 servings

- **1 can (12 ounces) pink salmon, undrained**
- **1 egg, lightly beaten**
- **¼ cup minced green onions**
- **1 tablespoon chopped fresh dill**
- **½ garlic powder**
- **½ cup rice flour**
- **1½ teaspoons baking powder**

1. Drain salmon, reserving 2 tablespoons liquid. Place salmon in medium bowl; break apart with fork. Add reserved liquid, egg, green onions, dill and garlic powder; mix well.
2. Combine rice flour and baking powder in small bowl. Add to salmon mixture; mix well. Shape into six patties.
3. Spray large heavy skillet with nonstick cooking spray; heat over medium-high heat.
4. Add salmon patties; cook until golden brown, turning once. Remove from skillet with slotted spoon; drain on paper towels. Serve immediately.

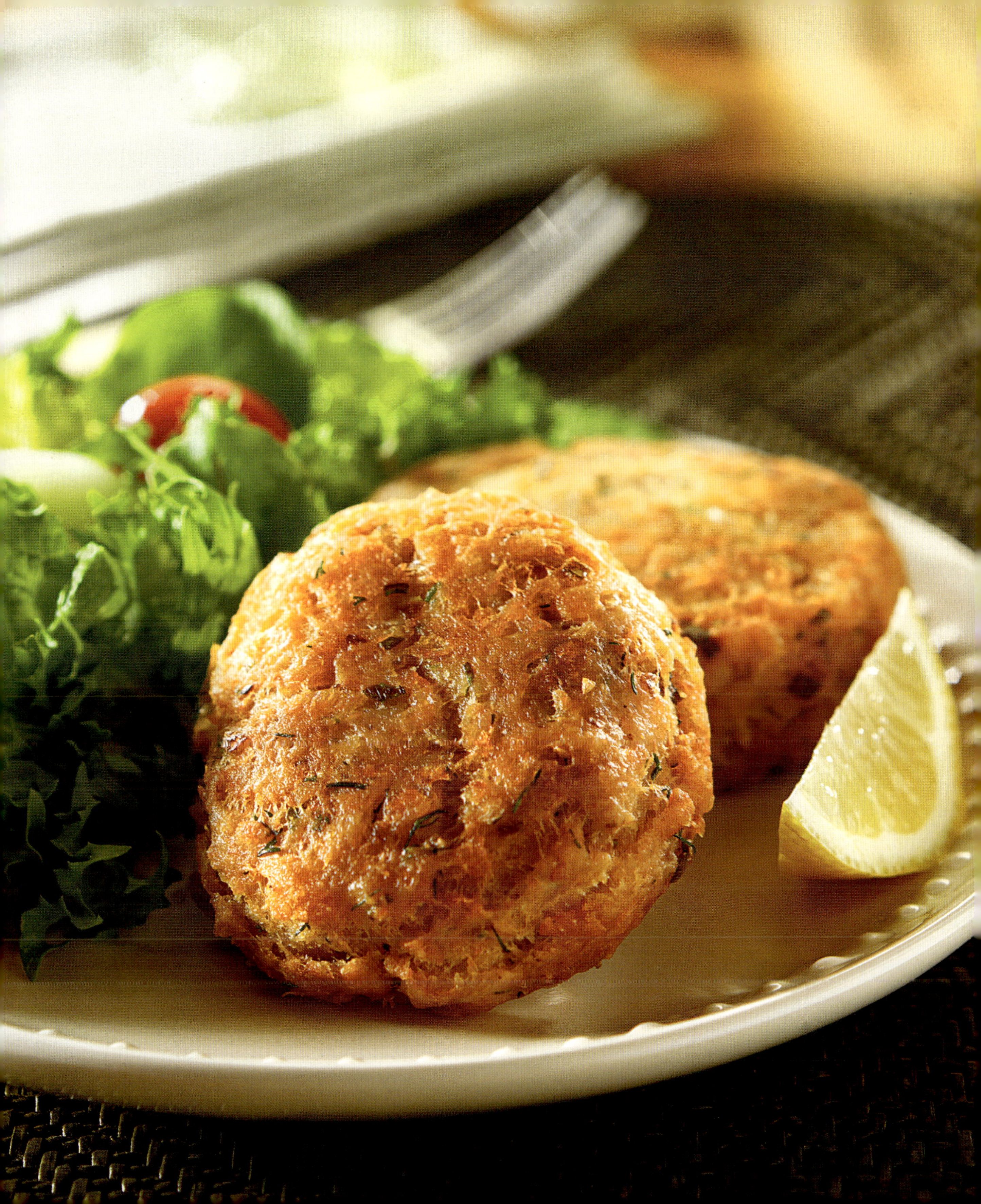

Pan-Cooked Bok Choy Salmon

makes 2 servings

- 1 pound bok choy or napa cabbage, chopped
- 1 cup broccoli slaw mix
- 2 tablespoons olive oil, divided
- 2 salmon fillets (4 to 6 ounces each)
- ¼ teaspoon salt
- ½ teaspoon black pepper
- 1 teaspoon sesame seeds

1. Combine bok choy and broccoli slaw mix in colander; rinse and drain well.
2. Heat 1 tablespoon oil in large nonstick skillet over medium heat. Sprinkle salmon with salt and pepper. Add salmon to skillet; cook about 3 minutes per side. Remove to plate.
3. Add remaining 1 tablespoon oil and sesame seeds to skillet; stir to toast sesame seeds. Add bok choy mixture; cook and stir 3 to 4 minutes.
4. Return salmon to skillet. Reduce heat to low; cover and cook about 4 minutes or until salmon begins to flake when tested with fork. Season with additional salt and pepper, if desired.

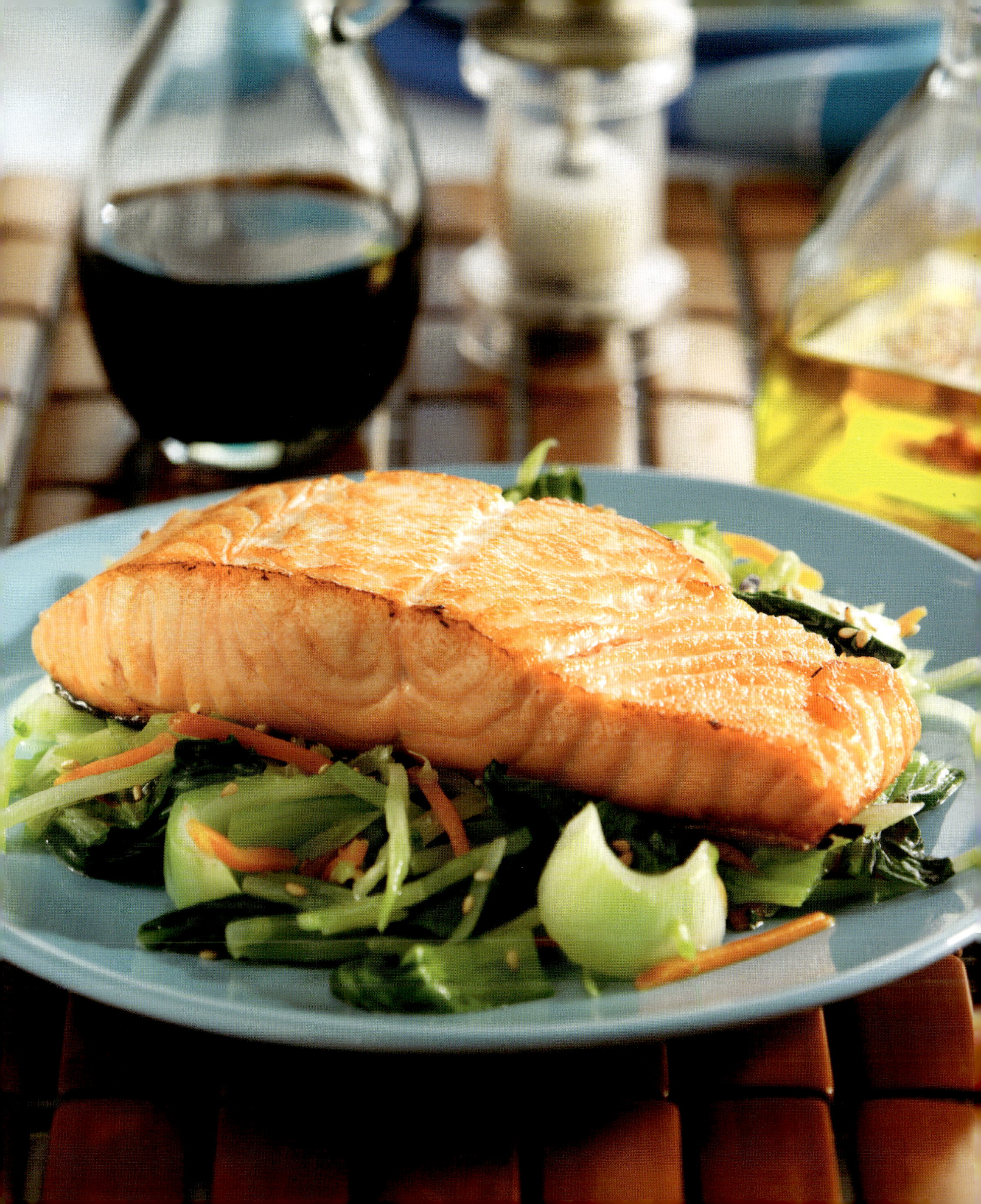

Tilapia with Spinach and Feta

makes 2 servings

- 1 teaspoon olive oil
- 4 cups baby spinach
- 2 skinless tilapia fillets or other mild white fish (4 ounces each)
- ½ teaspoon garlic powder
- ¼ teaspoon black pepper
- 2 ounces reduced-fat feta cheese, cut into 2 (3-inch) pieces

1. Preheat oven to 350°F. Spray baking sheet with nonstick cooking spray.
2. Heat oil in medium skillet over medium-low heat. Add spinach; cook just until wilted, stirring occasionally.
3. Arrange tilapia on prepared baking sheet; sprinkle with garlic powder and pepper. Place one piece of cheese on each fillet; top with spinach mixture.
4. Fold one end of each fillet up and over filling; secure with toothpick. Repeat with opposite end of each fillet.
5. Bake 20 minutes or until fish begins to flake when tested with fork.

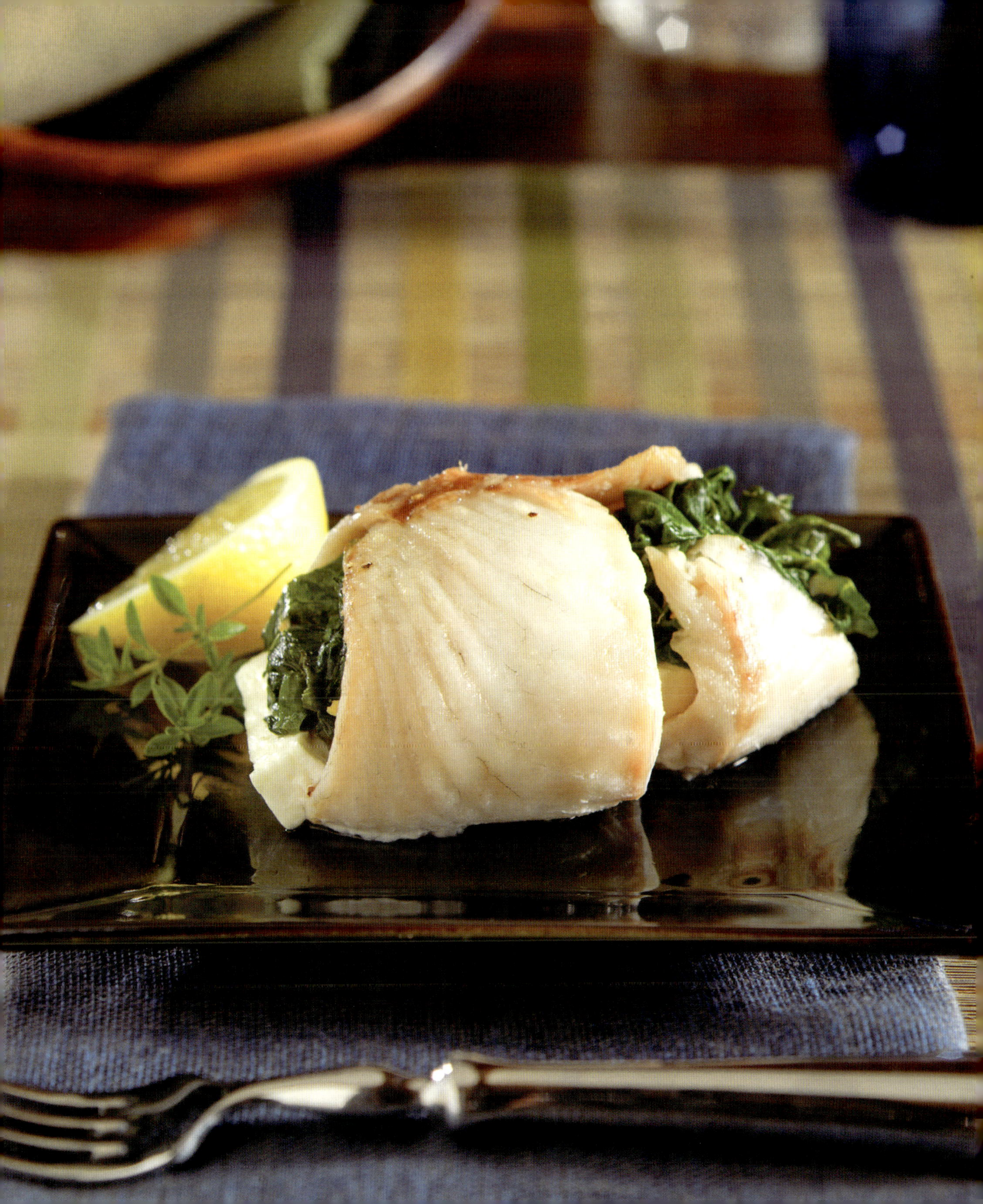

Shrimp and Tomato Salad

makes 4 servings

- 8 ounces cooked medium shrimp
- 1 cup cherry tomatoes, halved (or whole small yellow pear tomatoes)
- ¼ cup chopped or thinly sliced fresh basil leaves
- 1 tablespoon olive oil
- 1 tablespoon white wine vinegar
- ¼ teaspoon freshly ground black pepper
- 8 large Boston lettuce leaves
- ½ cup crumbled reduced-fat feta cheese (optional)

1. Combine shrimp, tomatoes, basil, oil, vinegar and pepper in medium bowl; mix well.
2. Serve over lettuce and top with cheese, if desired.

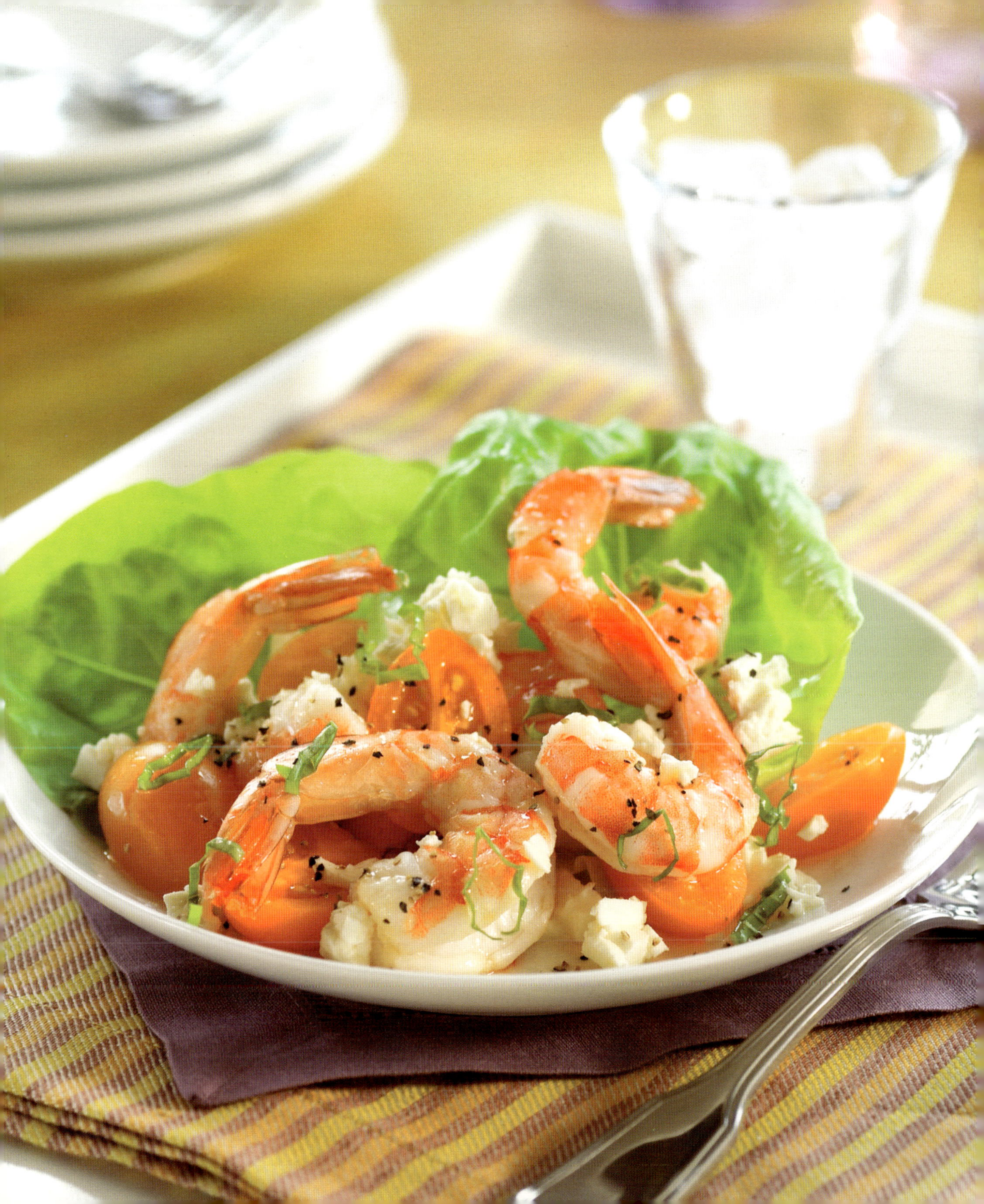

Sesame Peanut Spaghetti Squash

makes 4 servings

- 1 spaghetti squash (3 pounds)
- ⅓ cup sesame seeds
- ⅓ cup vegetable broth
- 2 tablespoons reduced-sodium soy sauce
- 1½ teaspoons sugar
- 2 teaspoons sesame oil
- 1 teaspoon cornstarch
- 1 teaspoon red pepper flakes
- 1 tablespoon vegetable oil
- 2 medium carrots, julienned
- 1 large red bell pepper, seeded and thinly sliced
- ¼ cup fresh snow peas, cut diagonally in half
- ½ cup coarsely chopped unsalted peanuts (optional)
- ⅓ cup minced fresh cilantro

1. Preheat oven to 350°F. Spray 13×9-inch baking dish with nonstick cooking spray. Cut squash in half lengthwise. Remove and discard seeds. Place squash, cut sides down, in prepared dish. Bake 45 minutes to 1 hour or until tender.
2. Using oven mitts to hold squash, remove spaghetti-like strands with fork. Place strands in large bowl; cover and keep warm.
3. Heat large skillet over medium-high heat. Add sesame seeds; cook and stir 45 seconds or until golden brown. Transfer to blender; add broth, soy sauce, sugar, sesame oil, cornstarch and red pepper flakes. Blend until mixture is coarsely puréed.
4. Heat oil in large skillet over medium-high heat 1 minute. Add carrots; cook and stir 1 minute. Add bell pepper; cook and stir 2 minutes or until vegetables are crisp-tender. Add snow peas; stir-fry 1 minute. Stir sesame seed mixture; add to wok. Cook and stir 1 minute or until sauce is thickened.
5. Serve sauce over spaghetti squash; top with peanuts, if desired, and cilantro.

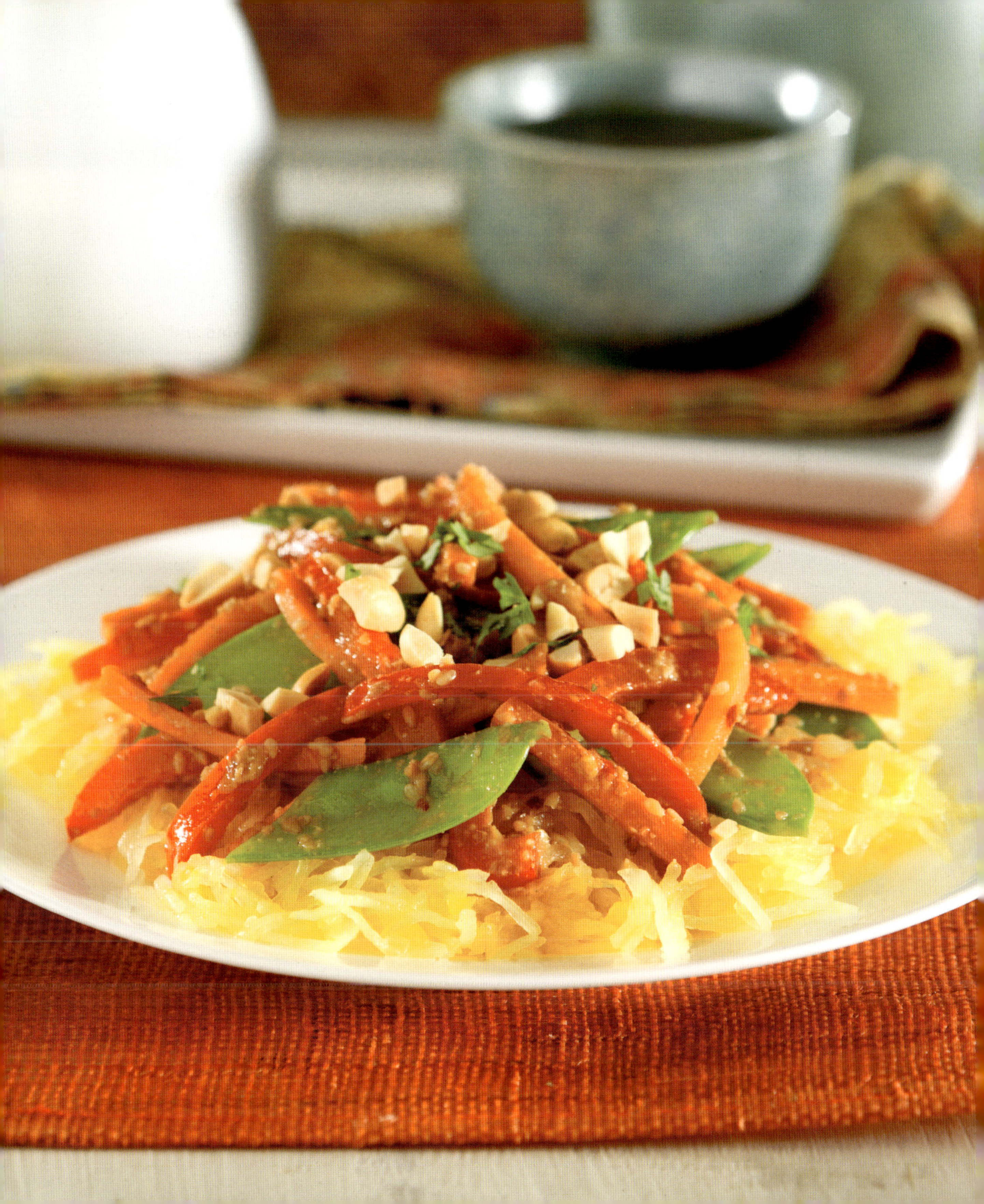

Lemon-Baked Fish with Cajun Buttery Topping

makes 4 servings

3 medium lemons, divided

4 tilapia fillets (about 1 pound total) rinsed and patted dry

½ teaspoon dried thyme

¼ teaspoon salt

¼ teaspoon black pepper

1 tablespoon butter

1 tablespoon hot pepper sauce (optional)

2 tablespoons chopped fresh parsley, divided

1. Preheat oven to 400°F. Line baking sheet with foil. Cut two lemons into four slices each. Arrange lemon slices in four rows of two slices each on prepared baking sheet. Place one fillet on top of each row.
2. Combine thyme, salt and pepper in small bowl; sprinkle evenly over fish. Bake 10 to 12 minutes or until fish is opaque in center.
3. Meanwhile, grate 2 teaspoons lemon peel from remaining lemon. Place in small bowl with butter, hot pepper sauce, if desired, and 1 tablespoon parsley; stir until well blended.
4. Top each fillet with sauce mixture; sprinkle with remaining 1 tablespoon parsley. Serve over lemon slices, if desired.

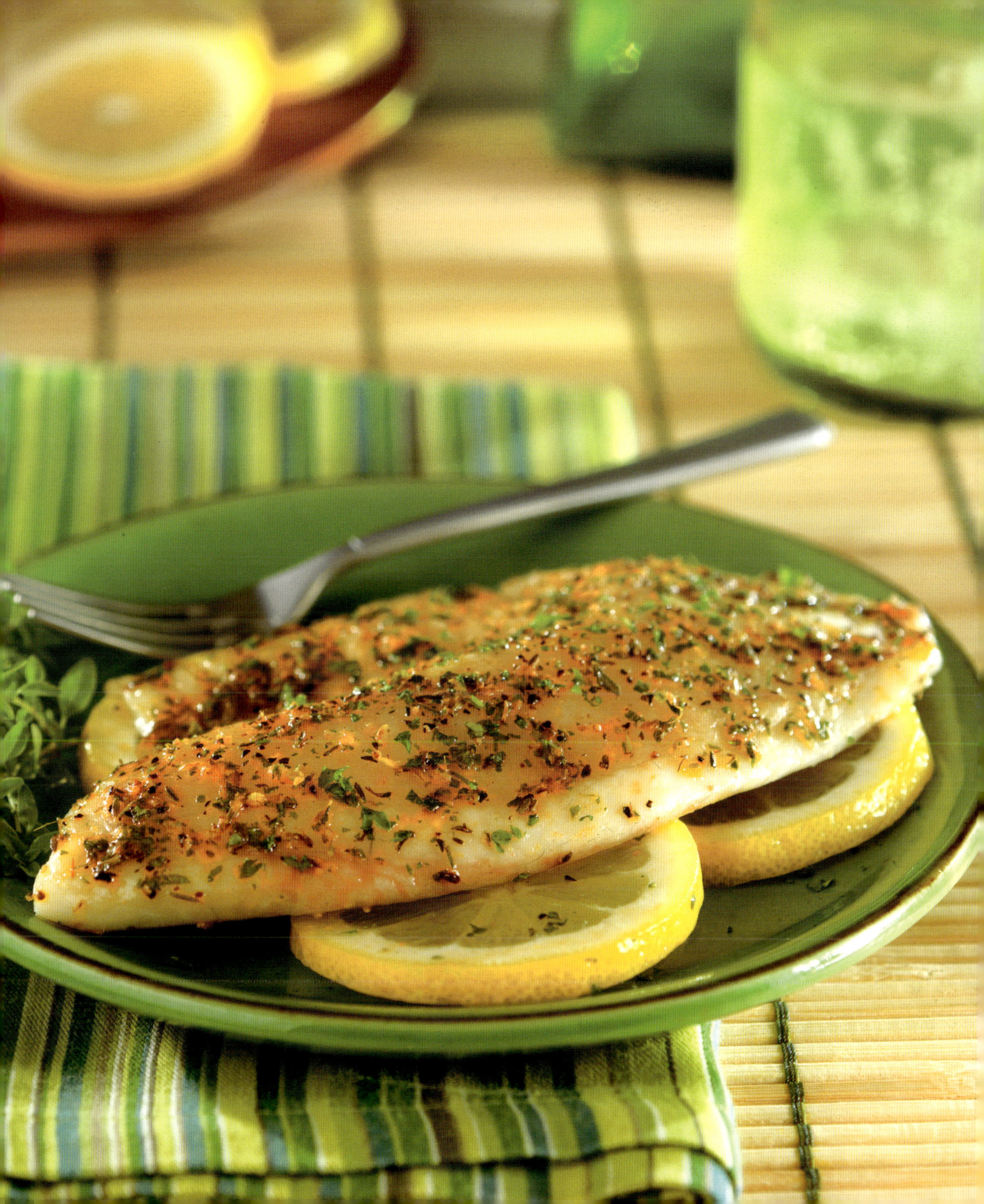

Szechuan Pork Stir-Fry over Spinach

makes 2 servings

- **2 teaspoons dark sesame oil, divided**
- **¾ cup matchstick carrots**
- **½ pound pork tenderloin, cut into thin strips**
- **2 teaspoons minced fresh ginger**
- **¼ teaspoon red pepper flakes**
- **1 tablespoon reduced-sodium soy sauce**
- **1 tablespoon mirin* or dry sherry**
- **2 teaspoons cornstarch**
- **8 ounces baby spinach**
- **2 teaspoons sesame seeds, toasted****

**Mirin, a sweet wine made from rice, is an essential flavoring in Japanese cuisine. It is available in Asian markets and the Asian or gourmet section of some supermarkets.*

***To toast sesame seeds, spread in small skillet. Shake skillet over medium-low heat about 3 minutes or until seeds begin to pop and turn golden.*

1. Heat 1 teaspoon oil in large nonstick skillet over medium-high heat. Add carrots; stir-fry 3 minutes. Add pork, ginger and red pepper flakes; stir-fry 3 minutes or until pork is barely pink in center.
2. Whisk soy sauce, mirin and cornstarch in small bowl until well blended. Pour into skillet; cook and stir 1 minute or until thickened.
3. Heat remaining 1 teaspoon oil in medium saucepan over medium-high heat. Add spinach; cover and cook 1 minute or until spinach is barely wilted.
4. Arrange spinach on two serving plates. Top with pork mixture; sprinkle with sesame seeds.

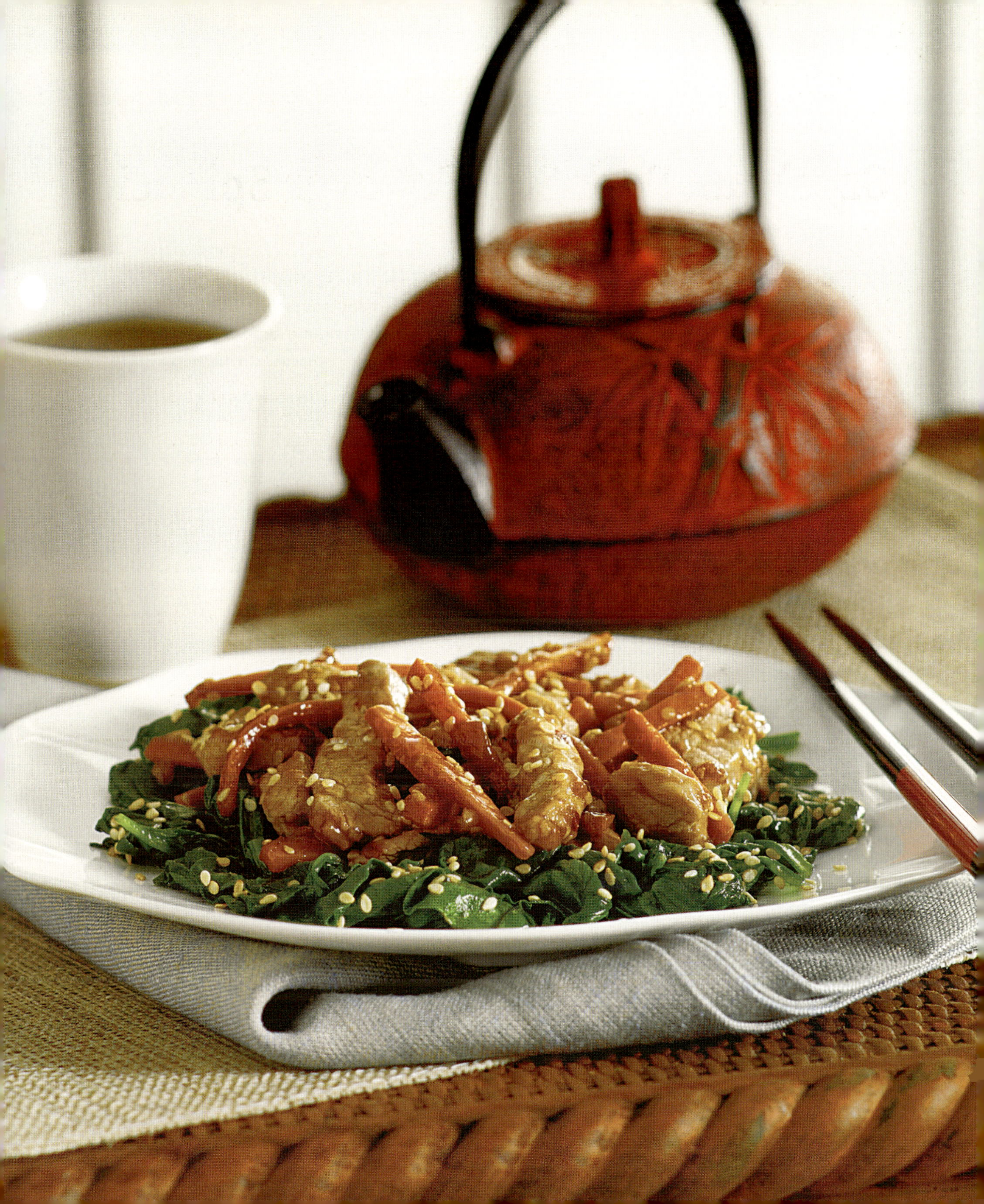

Vegetarian Stir-Fry

makes 4 servings

1 package (about 12 ounces) firm tofu
½ tablespoon salt-free seasoning blend
½ cup uncooked instant brown rice
1 bag (12 ounces) ready-to-use vegetable stir-fry mix
½ cup low-fat sesame ginger salad dressing

1. Preheat indoor grill or grill pan. Cut tofu into four 1-inch slices; sprinkle with seasoning blend.
2. Grill tofu 5 to 6 minutes or until browned. Meanwhile, prepare rice according to package instructions, omitting salt and fat.
3. Cook vegetables in microwave according to package instructions. Combine vegetables and dressing in medium bowl; toss to coat.
4. Divide rice and vegetables among four plates. Top with tofu.

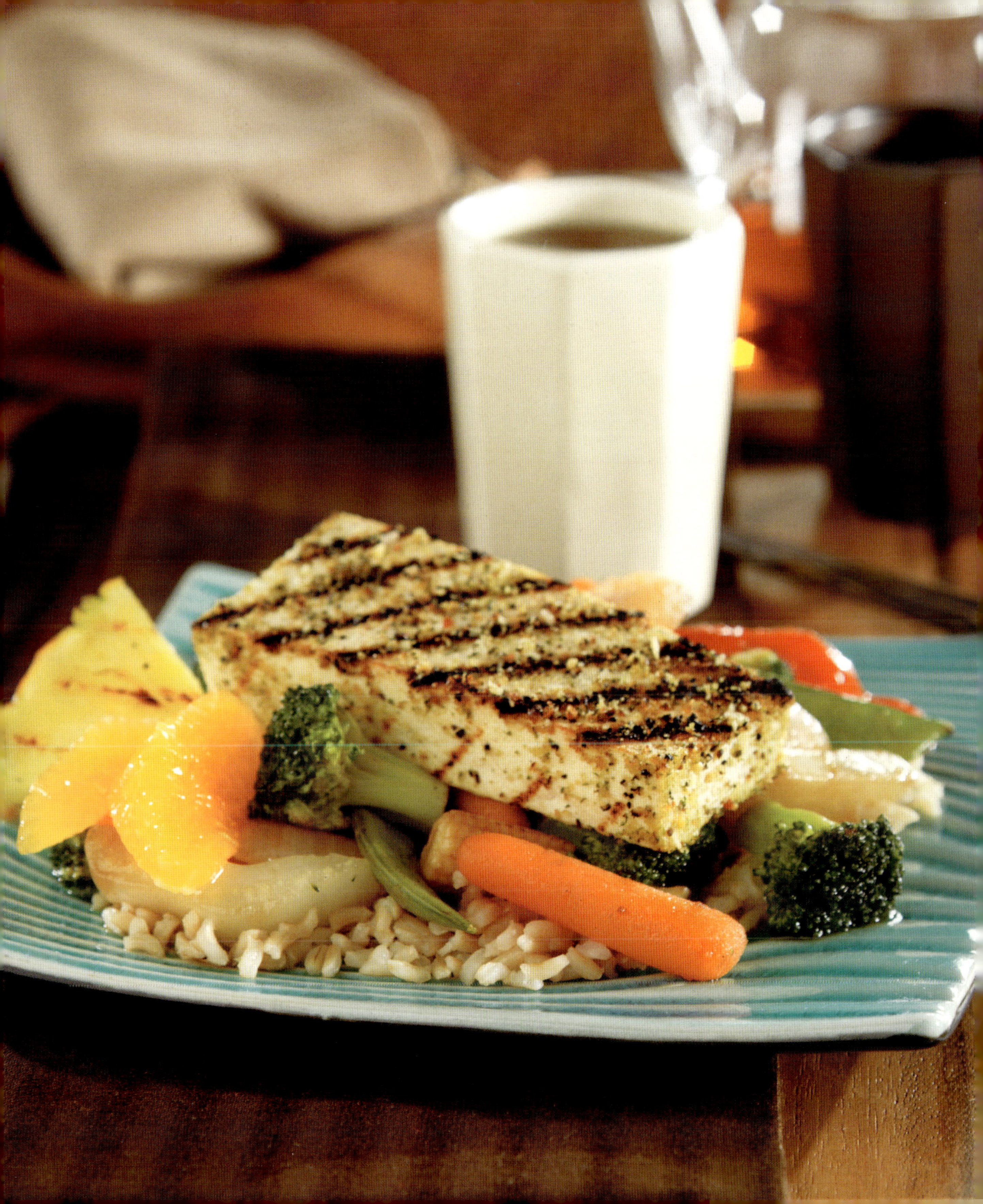

Scallops and Spinach over Potatoes

makes 4 servings

- **3 small or 2 medium Yukon Gold potatoes, cooked and diced**
- **12 ounces bay scallops, rinsed and patted dry**
- **¼ teaspoon salt**
- **¼ teaspoon black pepper**
- **4 cups baby spinach leaves**
- **2 tablespoons minced fresh chives**
- **1 teaspoon minced fresh tarragon**

1. Spray large heavy skillet with nonstick cooking spray; heat over medium-high heat. Add potatoes; cook 10 to 12 minutes or until browned, stirring occasionally. Remove to serving dish; keep warm.
2. Spray same skillet with cooking spray; heat over medium-high heat. Add scallops, salt and pepper; cook and stir 3 minutes or until scallops begin to give off liquid.
3. Add spinach, chives and tarragon. Reduce heat to medium; cook and stir 2 to 3 minutes or until scallops are cooked through and spinach is tender. Drain liquid from skillet. Spoon scallop mixture over potatoes; serve immediately.

TIP Fresh herbs are very perishable so purchase them in small amounts. For short-term storage, place the herb stems in water. Cover leaves loosely with a plastic bag or plastic wrap and store in the refrigerator. They will last from 2 days (basil, chives, dill, mint, oregano) to 5 days (rosemary, sage, tarragon, thyme).

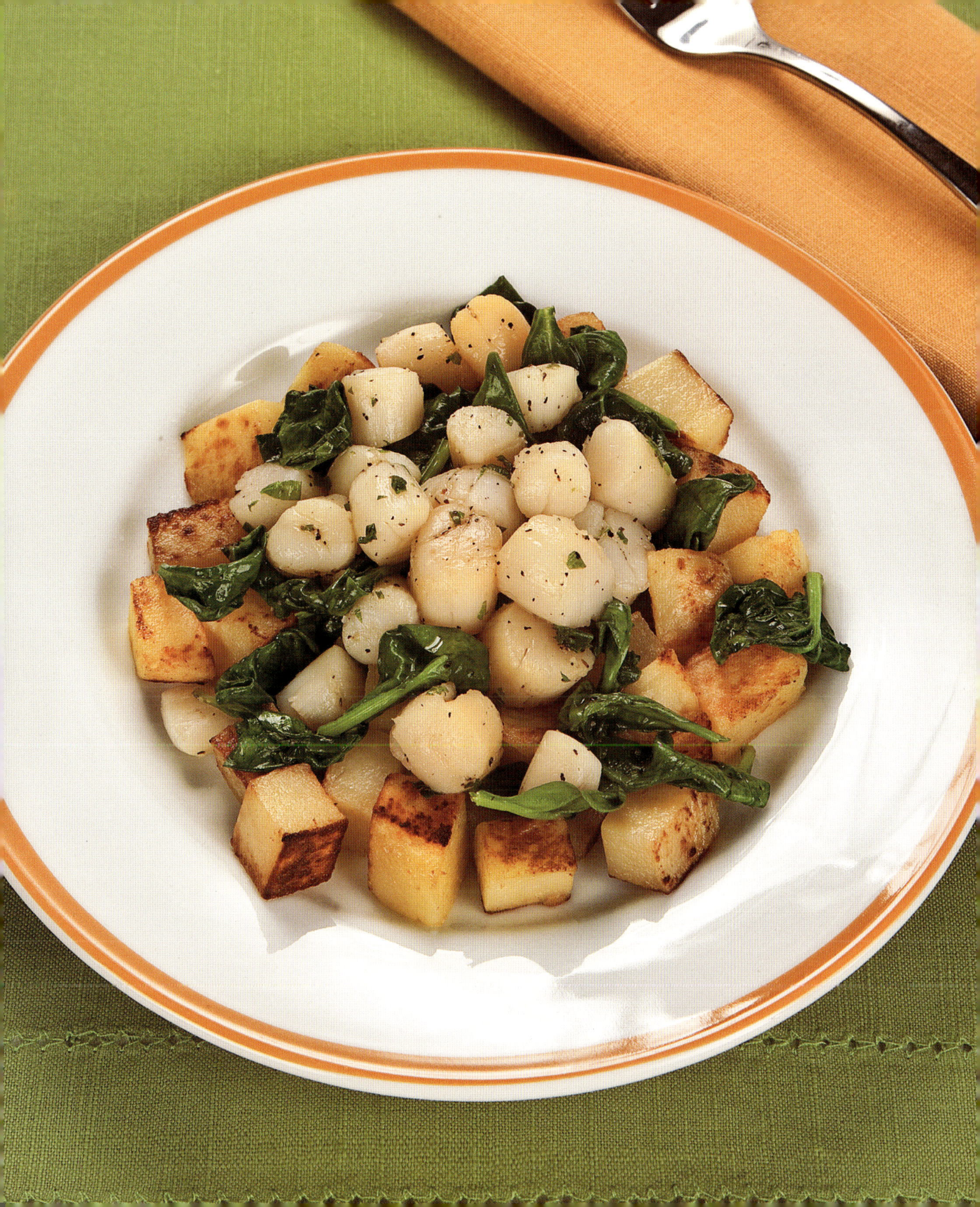

Szechuan Grilled Flank Steak

makes 4 to 6 servings

- **1 beef flank steak (1¼ to 1½ pounds)**
- **¼ cup seasoned rice wine vinegar**
- **¼ cup soy sauce**
- **2 tablespoons dark sesame oil**
- **2 teaspoons minced fresh ginger**
- **½ teaspoon garlic powder**
- **½ teaspoon red pepper flakes**
- **¼ cup water**
- **½ cup thinly sliced green onions (green parts only)**
- **2 to 3 teaspoons sesame seeds, toasted**
- **Hot cooked brown rice (optional)**

1. Place steak in large resealable food storage bag. Combine vinegar, soy sauce, oil, ginger, garlic powder and red pepper flakes in small bowl; pour over steak. Seal bag; turn to coat. Marinate in refrigerator 3 hours, turning once.
2. Prepare grill for direct cooking. Remove steak from marinade; reserve marinade in small saucepan. Grill steak, uncovered, over medium heat 17 to 21 minutes for medium rare to medium or to desired doneness, turning once. Transfer steak to cutting board; tent with foil and let stand 10 minutes.
3. Add water to reserved marinade. Bring to a rolling boil over high heat. Boil 1 minute.
4. Slice steak into thin slices against the grain. Drizzle with boiled marinade; sprinkle with green onions and sesame seeds. Serve with rice, if desired.

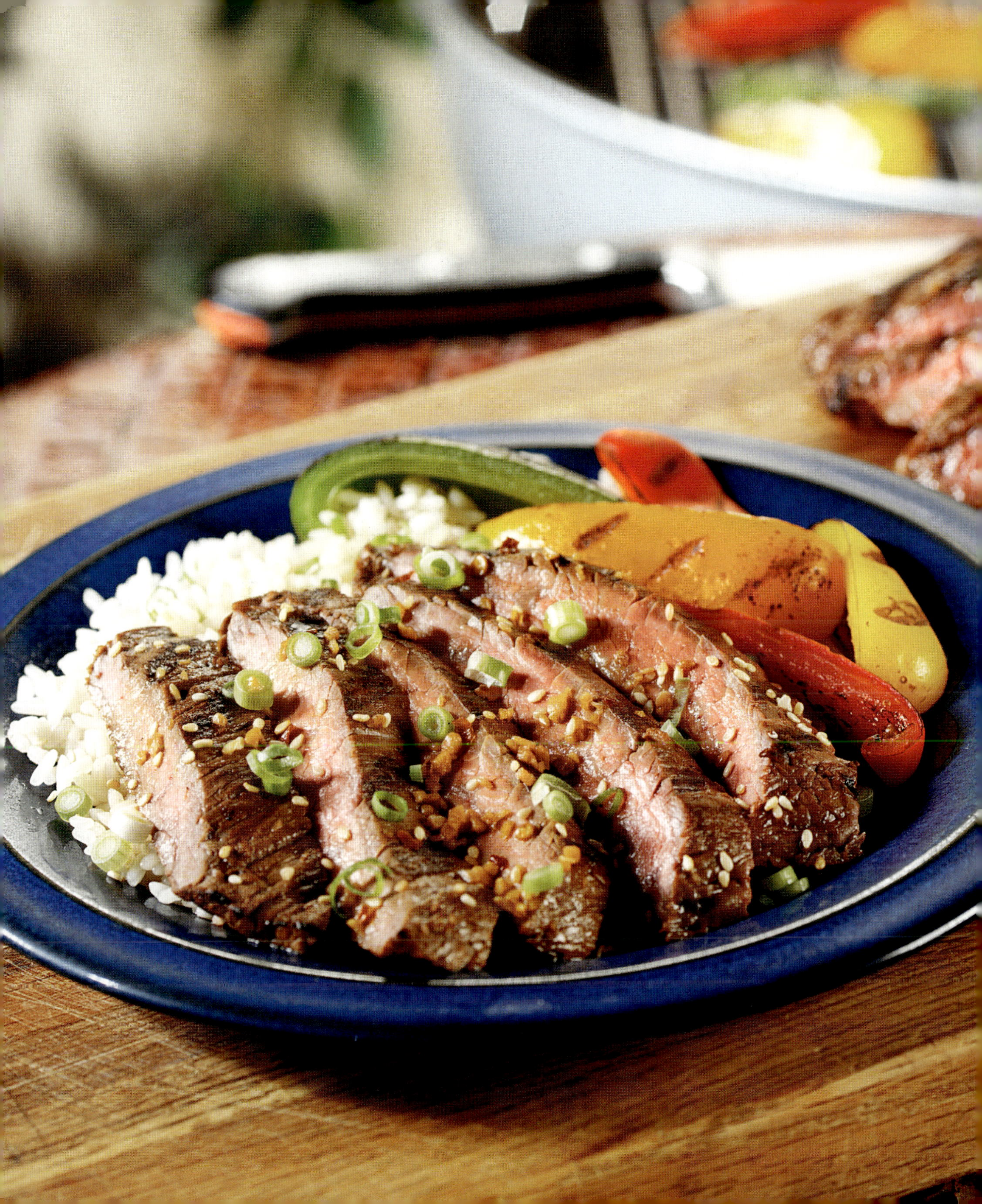

Tofu, Vegetable and Curry Stir-Fry

makes 4 servings

- **1 package (about 14 ounces) extra firm tofu, cut into ¾-inch cubes**
- **¾ cup unsweetened canned coconut milk**
- **2 tablespoons fresh lime juice**
- **1 tablespoon curry powder**
- **2 teaspoons dark sesame oil, divided**
- **4 cups broccoli florets (1½ inch pieces)**
- **2 medium red bell peppers, cut into short, thin strips**
- **¼ teaspoon salt**
- **Hot cooked brown rice (optional)**

1. Press tofu cubes between layers of paper towels to remove excess moisture. Combine coconut milk, lime juice and curry powder in medium bowl.
2. Heat 1 teaspoon oil in large nonstick skillet over medium heat. Add tofu; cook 10 minutes or until lightly browned on all sides, turning frequently. Remove to plate; set aside.
3. Add remaining 1 teaspoon oil to skillet; increase heat to high. Add broccoli and bell peppers; stir-fry about 5 minutes or until vegetables are crisp-tender.
4. Stir in tofu and coconut milk mixture; cook and stir until mixture comes to a boil. Stir in salt. Serve immediately with rice, if desired.

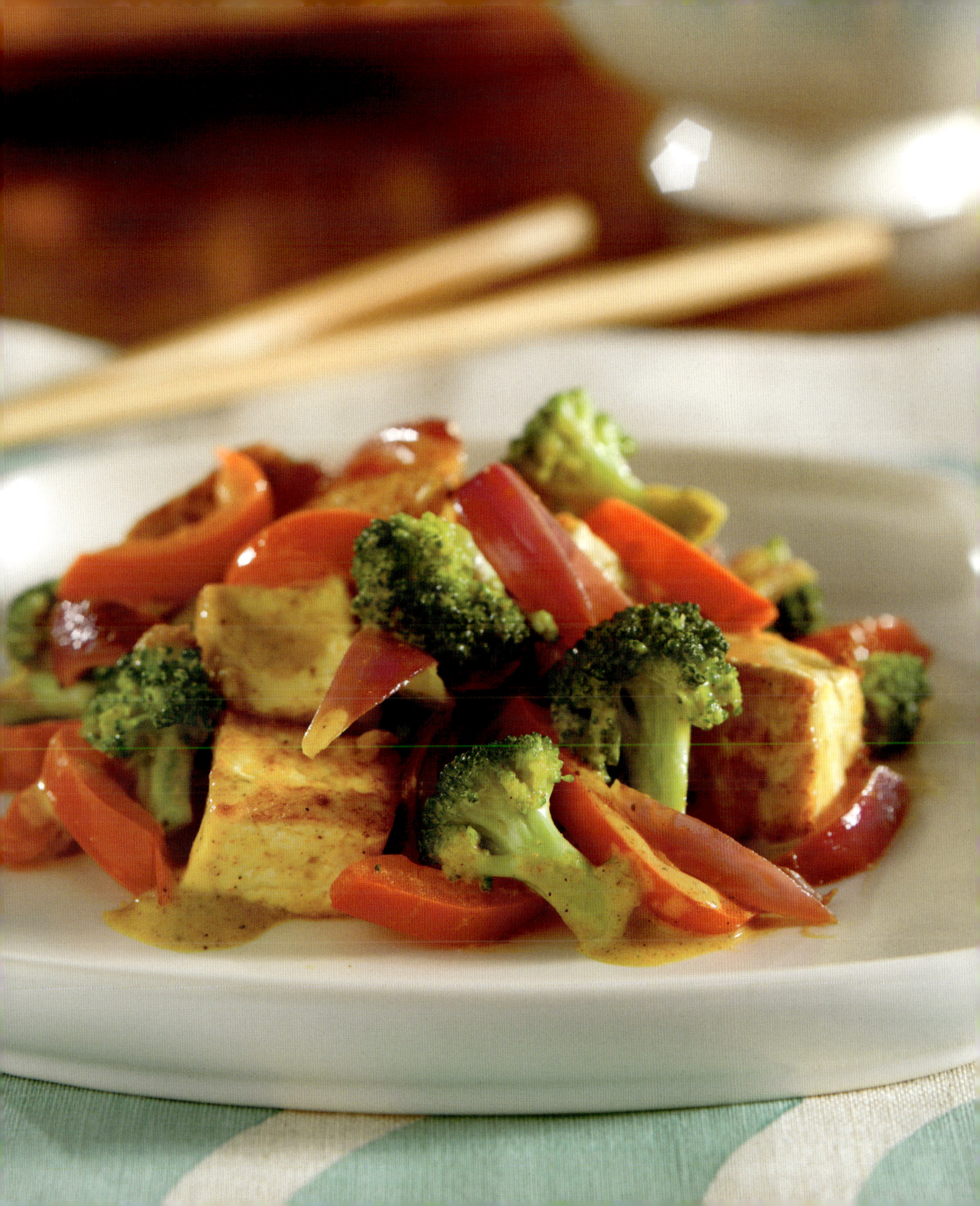

Miso Salmon and Spinach

makes 4 servings

½ cup sake

¼ cup white miso*

¼ cup mirin

4 boneless skinless salmon fillets or steaks (about 5 ounces each)

1 bag (10 ounces) baby spinach

Soy sauce

2 teaspoons sesame seeds, toasted

***Miso is a fermented soybean paste used frequently in Japanese cooking. It comes in many varieties; the light yellow miso, usually labeled "white" is the mildest. Look for it in tubs or plastic pouches in the produce section or Asian aisle of the supermarket.**

1. Combine sake, miso and mirin in large deep skillet or Dutch oven; bring to a boil over high heat. Reduce heat to medium; add salmon. Simmer, uncovered, 4 minutes. Turn salmon; simmer 3 to 4 minutes or until salmon is opaque in center. Transfer salmon to plate and keep warm.
2. Add spinach to liquid in skillet in two batches; cook 2 minutes or until spinach is wilted. Remove spinach to medium bowl with slotted spoon; cover to keep warm.
3. Turn heat to high and bring liquid to a gentle boil. Cook 1 to 2 minutes or until sauce is reduced to about ¼ cup. Season with soy sauce.
4. Serve salmon over spinach; drizzle with sauce and sprinkle with sesame seeds.

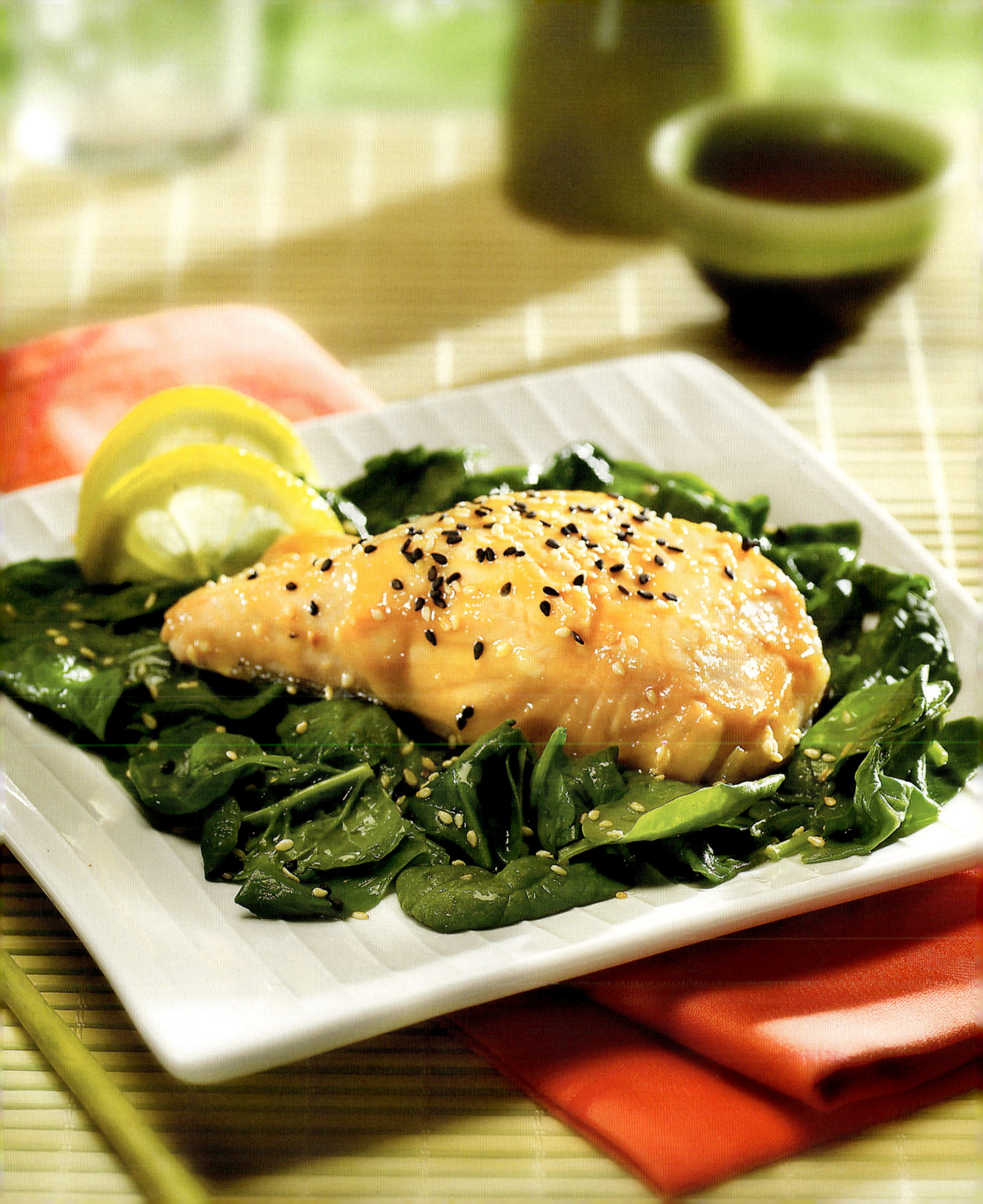

Noodles with Baby Shrimp

makes 4 to 6 servings

- **1 package (3¾ ounces) cellophane noodles**
- **3 green onions**
- **1 tablespoon olive oil**
- **1 package (16 ounces) frozen mixed vegetables (such as cauliflower, broccoli and carrots)**
- **1 cup vegetable broth**
- **8 ounces cooked frozen baby shrimp**
- **1 tablespoon soy sauce**
- **2 teaspoons dark sesame oil**
- **¼ teaspoon black pepper**

1. Place noodles in large bowl. Cover with boiling water; let stand 10 to 15 minutes or just until softened. Drain noodles. Cut noodles into 5- or 6-inch pieces; set aside. Cut green onions into 1-inch pieces.
2. Heat wok or large skillet over high heat about 1 minute or until hot. Drizzle olive oil into wok; heat 30 seconds. Add green onions; stir-fry 1 minute. Add mixed vegetables; stir-fry 2 minutes. Add broth; bring to a boil. Reduce heat to low; cover and cook 5 minutes or until vegetables are crisp-tender.
3. Add shrimp to wok; cook just until thawed. Stir in noodles, soy sauce, sesame oil and pepper; stir-fry until heated through.

TIP Cellophane noodles are also called bean thread noodles or glass noodles. These clear, thin noodles are made from mung bean starch so they are gluten-free. They are sold in packages of six to eight tangled bunches in the Asian section of the supermarket.

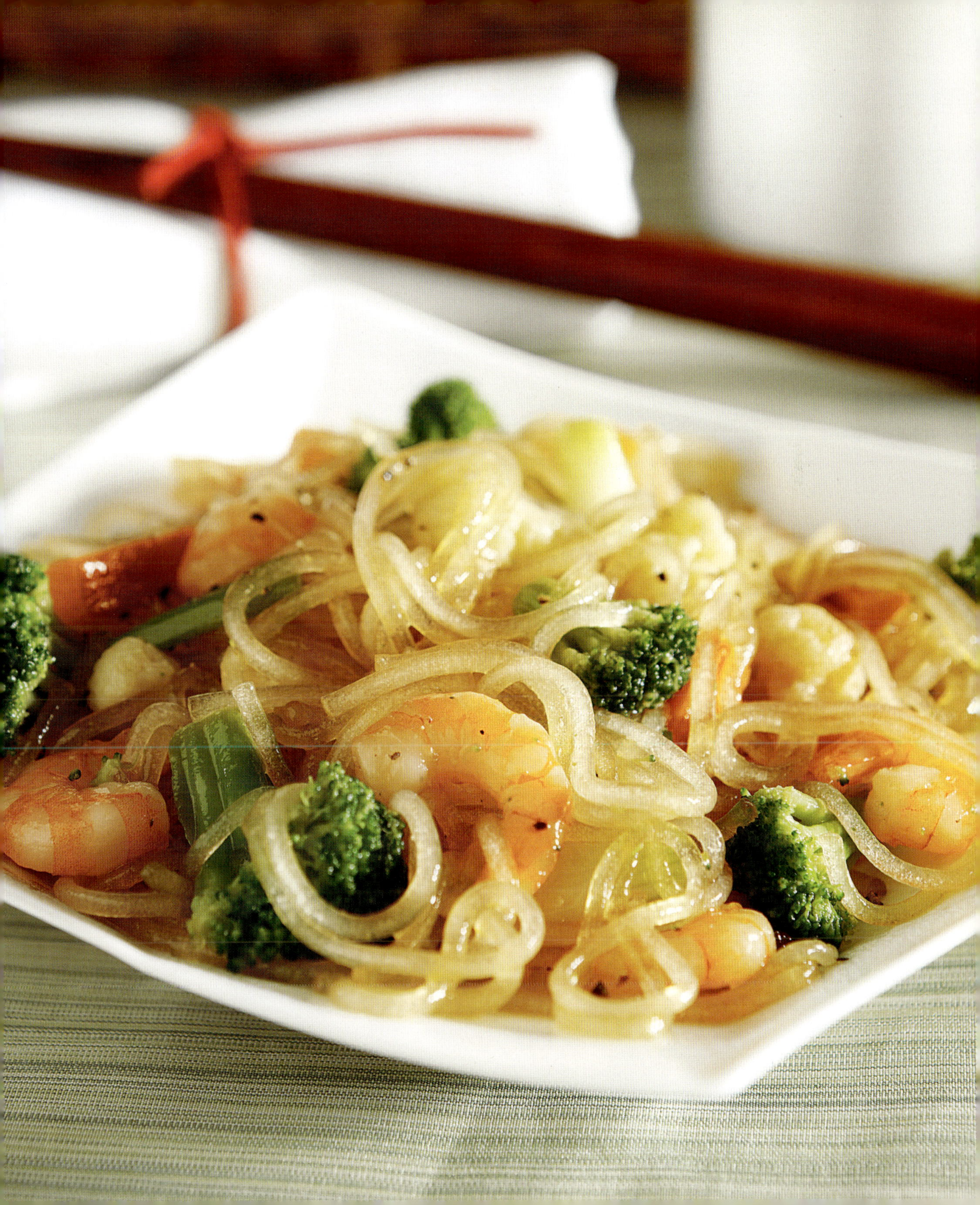

Pan-Seared Tuna with Spicy Horseradish Sauce

makes 4 servings

Spicy Horseradish Sauce

- ½ cup fat-free plain Greek yogurt
- 1 tablespoon water
- 2 teaspoons prepared horseradish
- 1 teaspoon Dijon mustard
- ½ teaspoon garlic powder
- ½ teaspoon dried rosemary
- ½ teaspoon salt
- 4 fresh tuna steaks (4 ounces each), rinsed and patted dry
- 2 teaspoons no-salt-added steak seasoning blend
- 2 tablespoons finely chopped parsley

1. Combine yogurt, water, horseradish, mustard, garlic powder, rosemary and salt in small bowl; set aside.
2. Sprinkle both sides of tuna with steak seasoning blend, pressing down with fingertips to adhere.
3. Spray grill pan with nonstick cooking spray; heat over medium-high heat. Cook tuna 1½ minutes on each side. (Do not overcook.) Remove to plates; top with parsley and horseradish sauce.

TIP Serve this recipe with green vegetables for a nutritious meal.

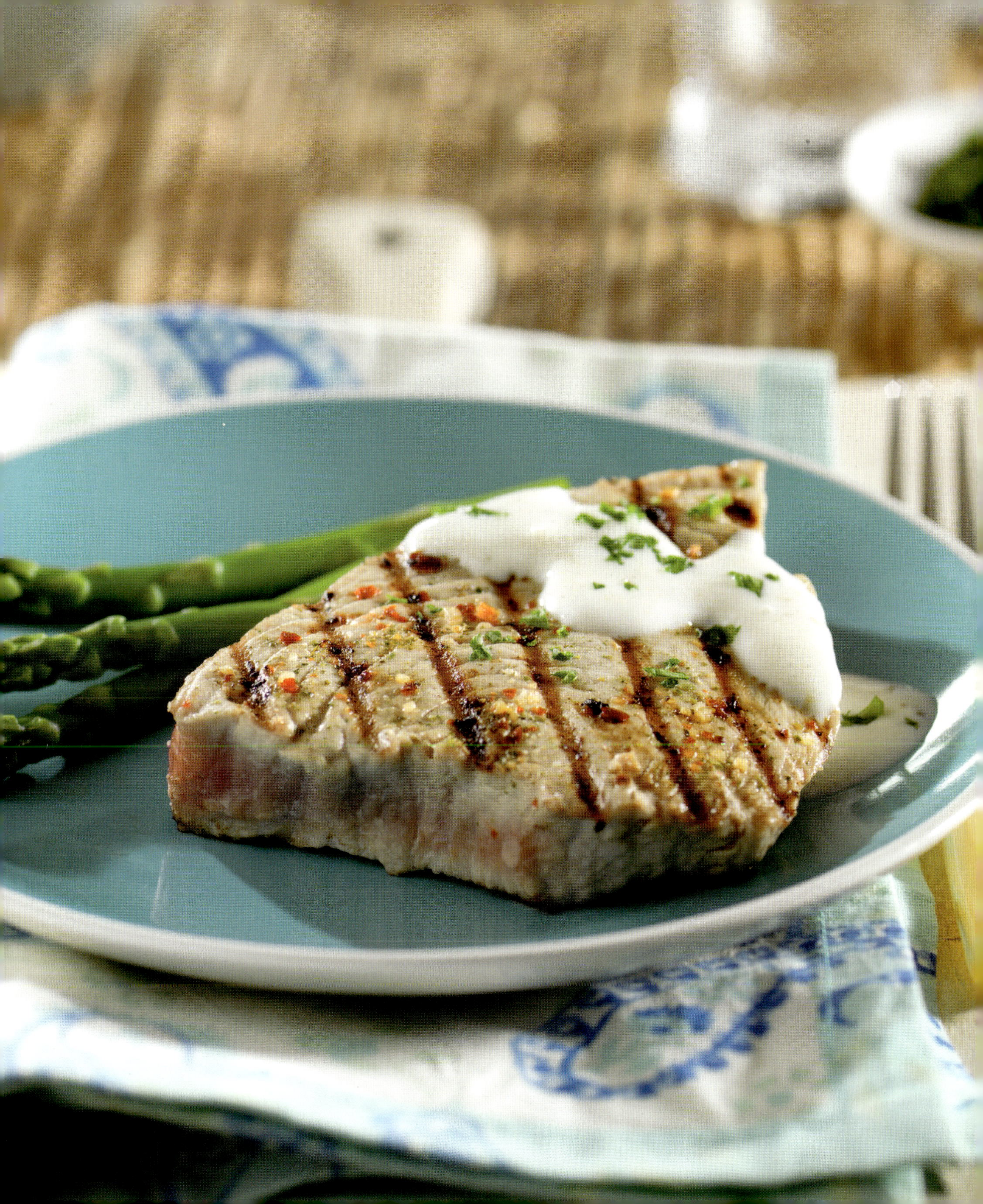

Shrimp and Veggie Skillet Toss

makes 4 servings

- ¼ cup soy sauce
- 2 tablespoons lime juice
- 1 tablespoon sesame oil
- 1 teaspoon grated fresh ginger
- ⅛ teaspoon red pepper flakes
- 32 medium raw shrimp (about 8 ounces total), peeled, deveined, rinsed and patted dry (with tails on)
- 2 medium zucchini, cut in half lengthwise and thinly sliced
- 6 green onions, trimmed and halved lengthwise
- 12 grape tomatoes

1. Whisk soy sauce, lime juice, oil, ginger and red pepper flakes in small bowl; set aside.
2. Spray large nonstick skillet with nonstick cooking spray; heat over medium-high heat. Add shrimp; cook and stir 3 minutes or until shrimp are pink and opaque. Remove from skillet.
3. Spray same skillet with cooking spray. Add zucchini; cook and stir 4 to 6 minutes or just until crisp-tender. Add green onions and tomatoes; cook 1 to 2 minutes. Add shrimp, cook 1 minute. Transfer to large bowl.
4. Add soy sauce mixture to skillet; bring to a boil. Remove from heat. Stir in shrimp and vegetables; gently toss to coat.

NOTE Shrimp are very low in calories and fat, and high in protein. They're also a good source of vitamin D and vitamin B12.

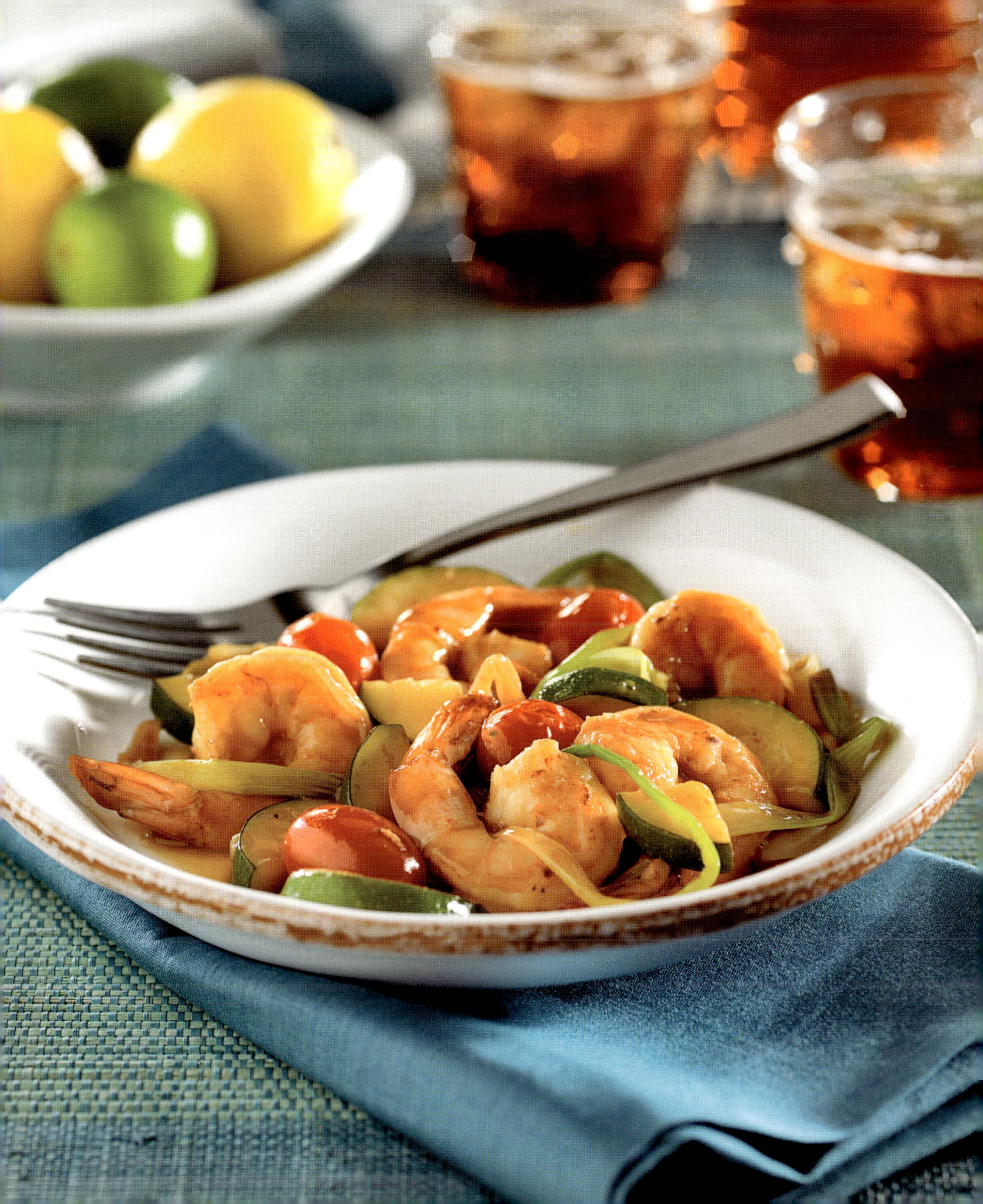

Curried Shrimp and Vegetable Noodle Bowl

makes 2 servings

- **2 ounces thin rice noodles (rice vermicelli)**
- **1 teaspoon canola oil**
- **¾ cup broccoli**
- **¼ cup snow peas, diagonally halved**
- **4 ounces medium raw shrimp, peeled and deveined**
- **1 cup packed chopped bok choy leaves**
- **⅓ cup unsweetened canned coconut milk**
- **1½ tablespoons red curry paste***
- **2 tablespoons chopped fresh cilantro**

****Red curry paste can be found in jars in the Asian food section of the supermarket. Spice levels can vary between brands. Start with 1 tablespoon, then add more as desired.***

1. Place rice noodles in medium bowl. Cover with hot water; let stand 15 minutes or until tender. Drain and cut noodles into 3-inch lengths.
2. Meanwhile, heat oil in large nonstick skillet over medium heat. Add broccoli and snow peas; stir-fry 3 minutes. Add shrimp and bok choy; stir-fry 5 minutes or until shrimp are pink and opaque and vegetables are crisp-tender. Add coconut milk and curry paste; stir-fry 1 to 2 minutes or until sauce is thickened.
3. Add noodles to skillet; toss to coat.
4. Divide mixture evenly among two bowls; sprinkle with cilantro.

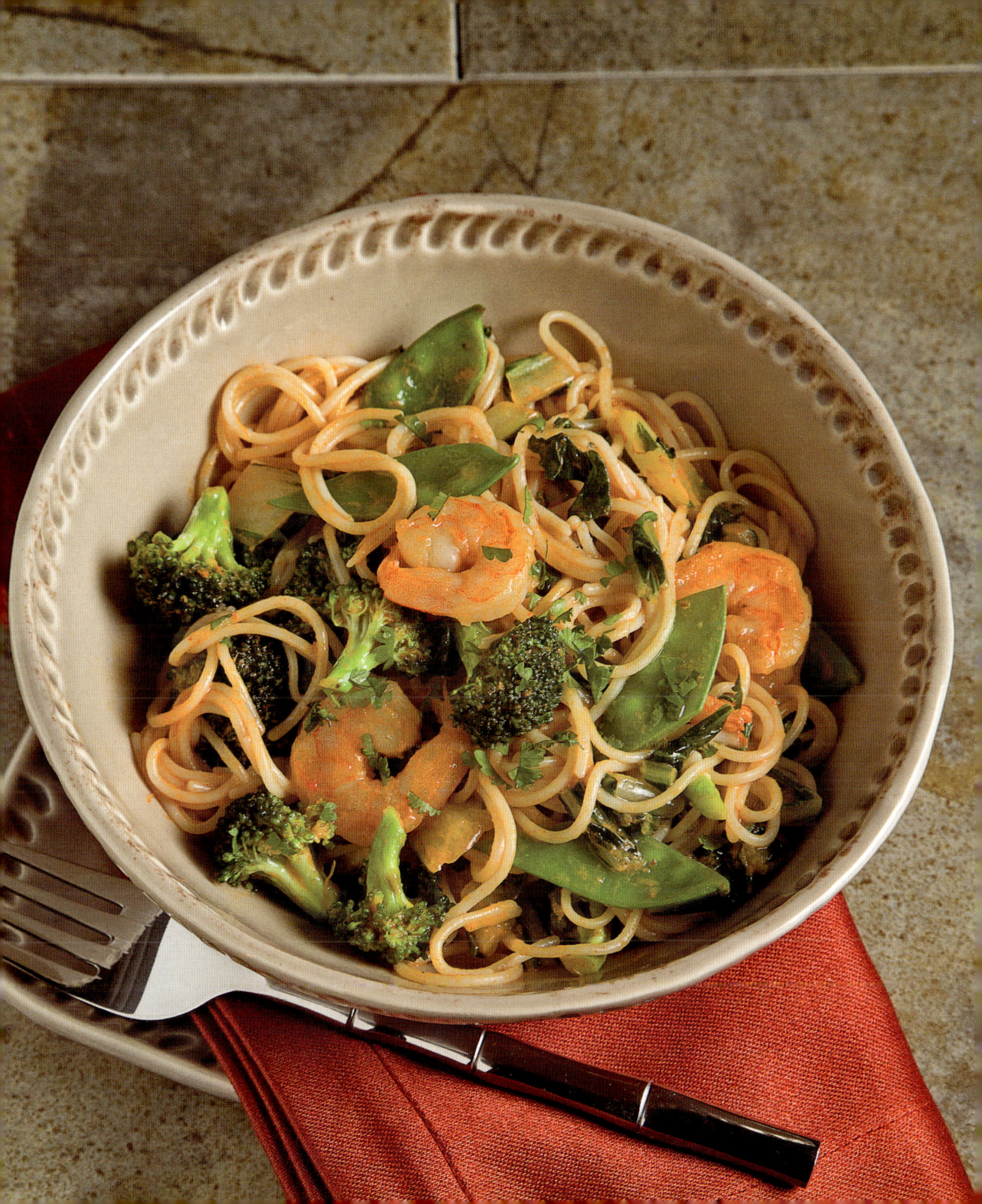

Sesame-Garlic Flank Steak

makes 4 servings

1 beef flank steak (about 1¼ pounds)
2 tablespoons soy sauce
2 tablespoons hoisin sauce
1 tablespoon dark sesame oil
½ teaspoon garlic powder

1. Score steak lightly with sharp knife in diamond pattern on both sides; place in large resealable food storage bag. Combine soy sauce, hoisin sauce, sesame oil and garlic powder in small bowl; pour over steak. Seal bag; turn to coat. Marinate in refrigerator at least 2 hours or up to 24 hours, turning once.
2. Prepare grill for direct cooking. Remove steak from marinade; reserve marinade.
3. Grill steak, covered, over medium heat 13 to 18 minutes for medium rare (130° to 135°F) or to desired doneness, turning and brushing with marinade halfway through cooking time. Discard remaining marinade.
4. Transfer steak to cutting board; tent with foil and let stand 10 minutes. Cut into thin slices across the grain.

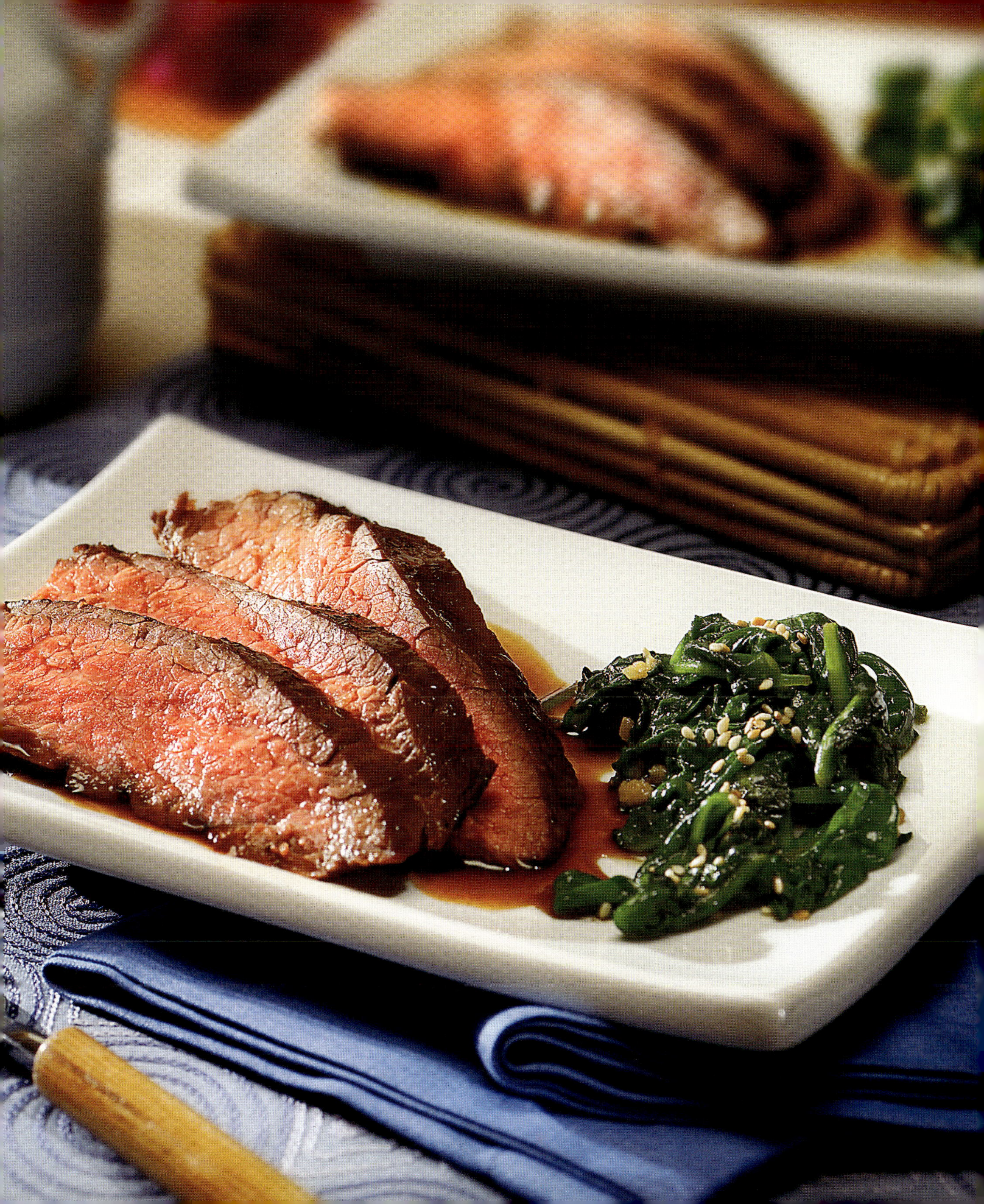

Shrimp, Chicken and Cucumber Salad

makes 4 servings

- 1 quart plus 3 tablespoons water, divided
- 3 chicken thighs (about 14 ounces)
- 2 medium cucumbers, cut in half lengthwise, seeded and thinly sliced
- 1 large carrot, cut into matchstick-size strips
- 1 teaspoon salt
- 2 tablespoons fish sauce
- 1 tablespoon sugar
- 1½ tablespoons fresh lime juice
- ½ teaspoon garlic powder
- 4 jumbo cooked shrimp, peeled and deveined (with tails on)
- 1 tablespoon chopped fresh cilantro
- 1 tablespoon chopped fresh mint
- 1 tablespoon chopped fresh basil
- 1 tablespoon chopped green onion

1. Heat 1 quart water in medium saucepan over high heat to boiling. Add chicken. Reduce heat to low; simmer, covered, until tender, about 25 minutes. Drain chicken; let stand until cool enough to handle. Skin and debone chicken; cut into ¼-inch pieces.
2. Meanwhile, combine cucumbers and carrot in large bowl; sprinkle with salt. Mix well; let stand 15 minutes.
3. For dressing, combine remaining 3 tablespoons water, fish sauce, sugar, lime juice and garlic powder in small bowl; stir until sugar is dissolved.
4. Squeeze cucumber mixture to extract liquid; discard liquid. Combine cucumber mixture and chicken in medium bowl; drizzle with dressing and toss to coat. Cover and refrigerate 30 minutes to 2 hours.
5. Cut shrimp in half lengthwise, leaving tails attached. Mix cilantro, mint, basil and green onion in small bowl.
6. Transfer salad mixture to serving bowl. Garnish with shrimp; top with mixed herbs.

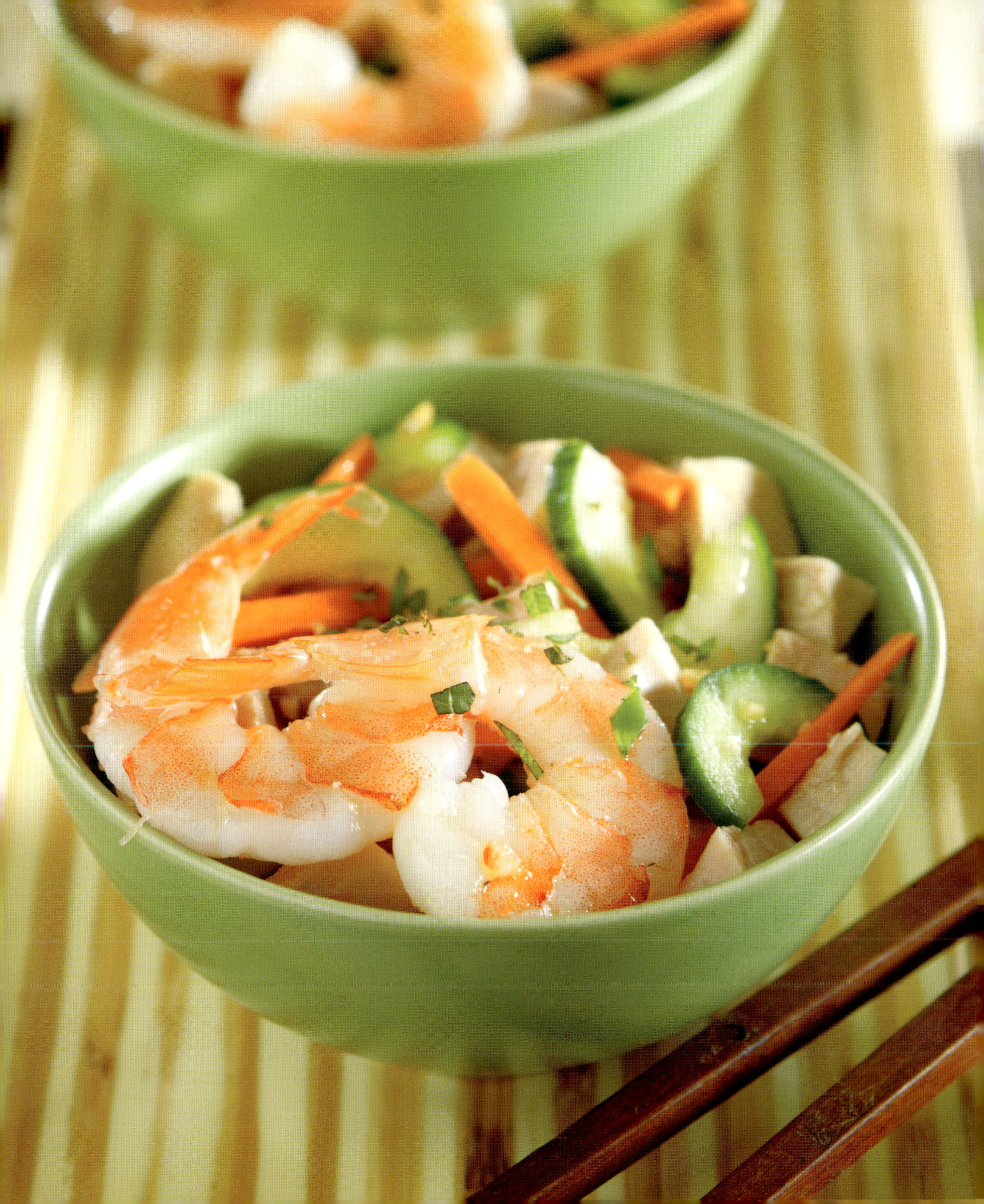

Herbed Lamb Chops

makes 4 to 6 servings

- ⅓ cup vegetable oil
- ⅓ cup red wine vinegar
- 2 tablespoons soy sauce
- 1 tablespoon lemon juice
- 1 teaspoon salt
- 1 teaspoon chopped fresh oregano *or* ¼ teaspoon dried oregano
- 1 teaspoon dried rosemary
- 1 teaspoon ground mustard
- ½ teaspoon garlic powder
- ½ teaspoon white pepper
- 8 lamb loin chops, 1 inch thick (about 2 pounds)

1. Combine oil, vinegar, soy sauce, lemon juice, salt, oregano, rosemary, mustard, garlic powder and pepper in large resealable food storage bag.
2. Reserve ½ cup marinade in small bowl. Add lamb to remaining marinade; seal bag and turn to coat. Marinate in refrigerator at least 1 hour.
3. Prepare grill for direct cooking over medium-high heat. Remove lamb from marinade; discard marinade.
4. Grill lamb over medium-high heat 8 minutes or to desired doneness, turning once and basting often with reserved ½ cup marinade. Do not baste during last 5 minutes of cooking. Discard any remaining marinade.

HINT Substitute ¼ to ½ teaspoon dried herbs for each teaspoon of fresh herbs.

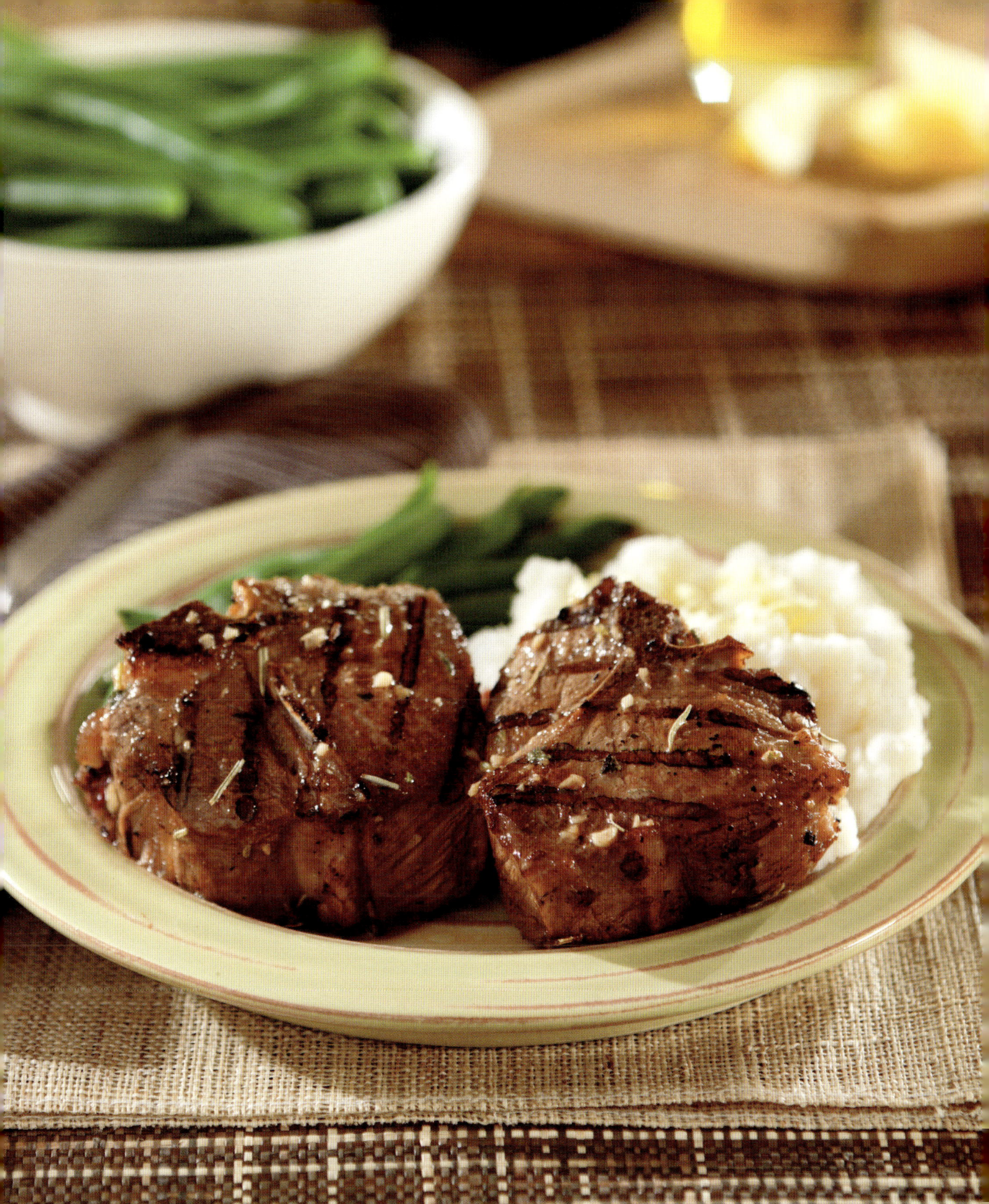

Hip Hop Hash

makes 4 servings

- 1 tablespoon olive oil
- 1 tablespoon sweet rice flour (mochiko)
- ⅓ cup beef broth
- 1 teaspoon Worcestershire sauce
- 1 pound cooked beef pot roast, diced
- 1 medium sweet potato (about 12 ounces), peeled and diced
- 1 stalk celery, diced
- ½ cup corn
- ¼ cup diced red or green bell pepper

1. Heat oil in large skillet over medium heat. Whisk in rice flour; cook 2 minutes, stirring constantly. Whisk in broth and Worcestershire sauce; bring to a simmer.
2. Add beef, sweet potato, celery, corn and bell pepper. Return to a simmer; cover and cook 12 minutes or until vegetables are tender.

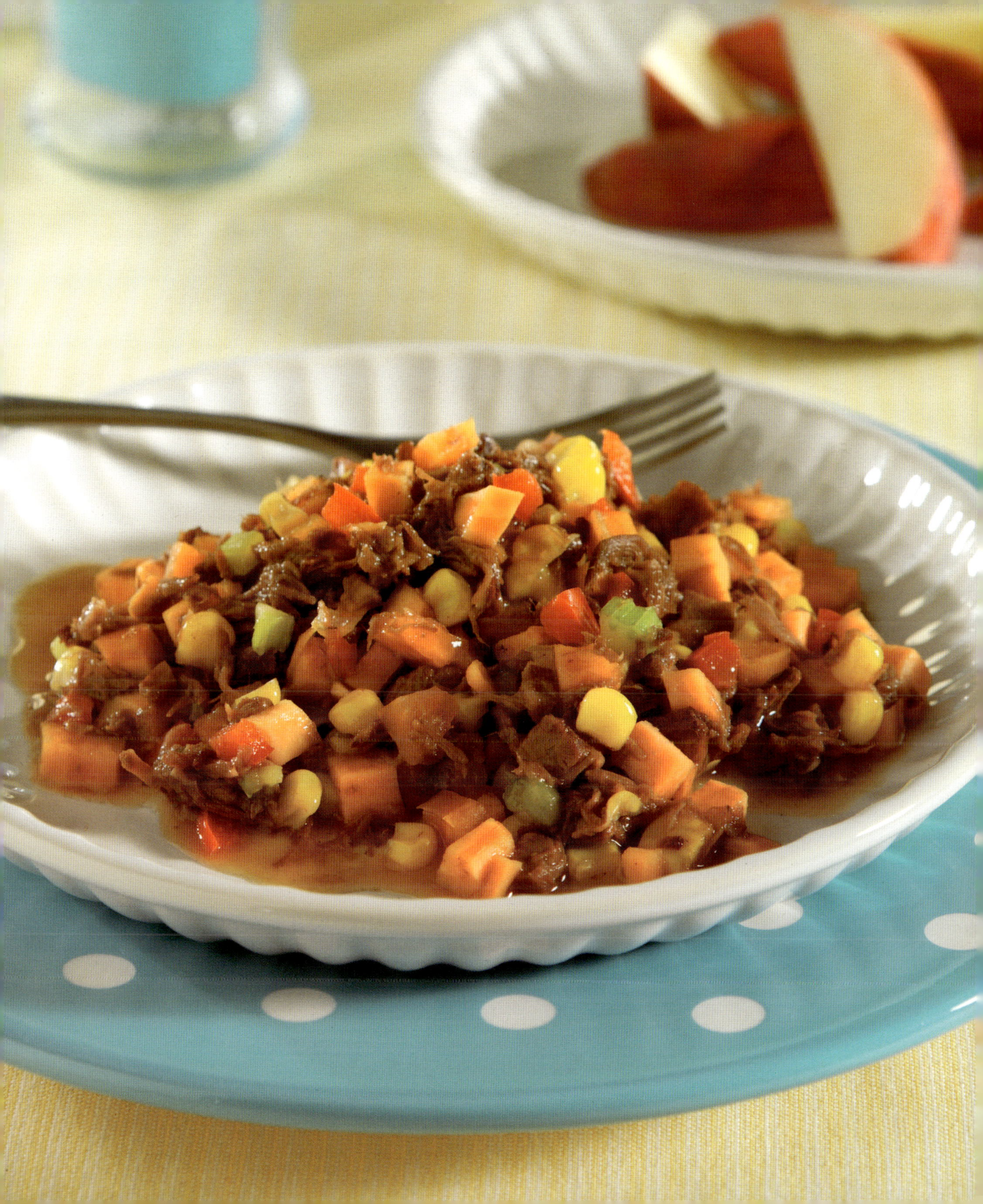

Chicken and Fruit Salad

makes 4 servings

- ¼ cup lemon juice
- 3 tablespoons olive oil
- 1½ tablespoons honey
- ½ teaspoon Dijon mustard
- ¼ teaspoon salt
- ⅛ teaspoon black pepper
- Pinch ground red pepper
- 8 cups mixed greens
- 2 grilled chicken breasts (4 to 6 ounces each), thinly sliced
- 1 cup sliced fresh strawberries
- ½ small mango, peeled and cut into thin 1-inch pieces
- ½ cup fresh blueberries
- ¼ cup thinly sliced red onion
- ¼ cup chopped walnuts

1. Combine lemon juice, oil, honey, mustard, salt, black pepper and red pepper in small bowl; whisk until well blended.
2. Divide greens among four serving plates. Top evenly with chicken, strawberries, mango, blueberries and onion. Drizzle with dressing; sprinkle with walnuts.

TIP You can swap out the fruit according to your taste and what's in season. Try using slices or chunks of apples, pears or plums and grapes in place of the fresh berries and mango.

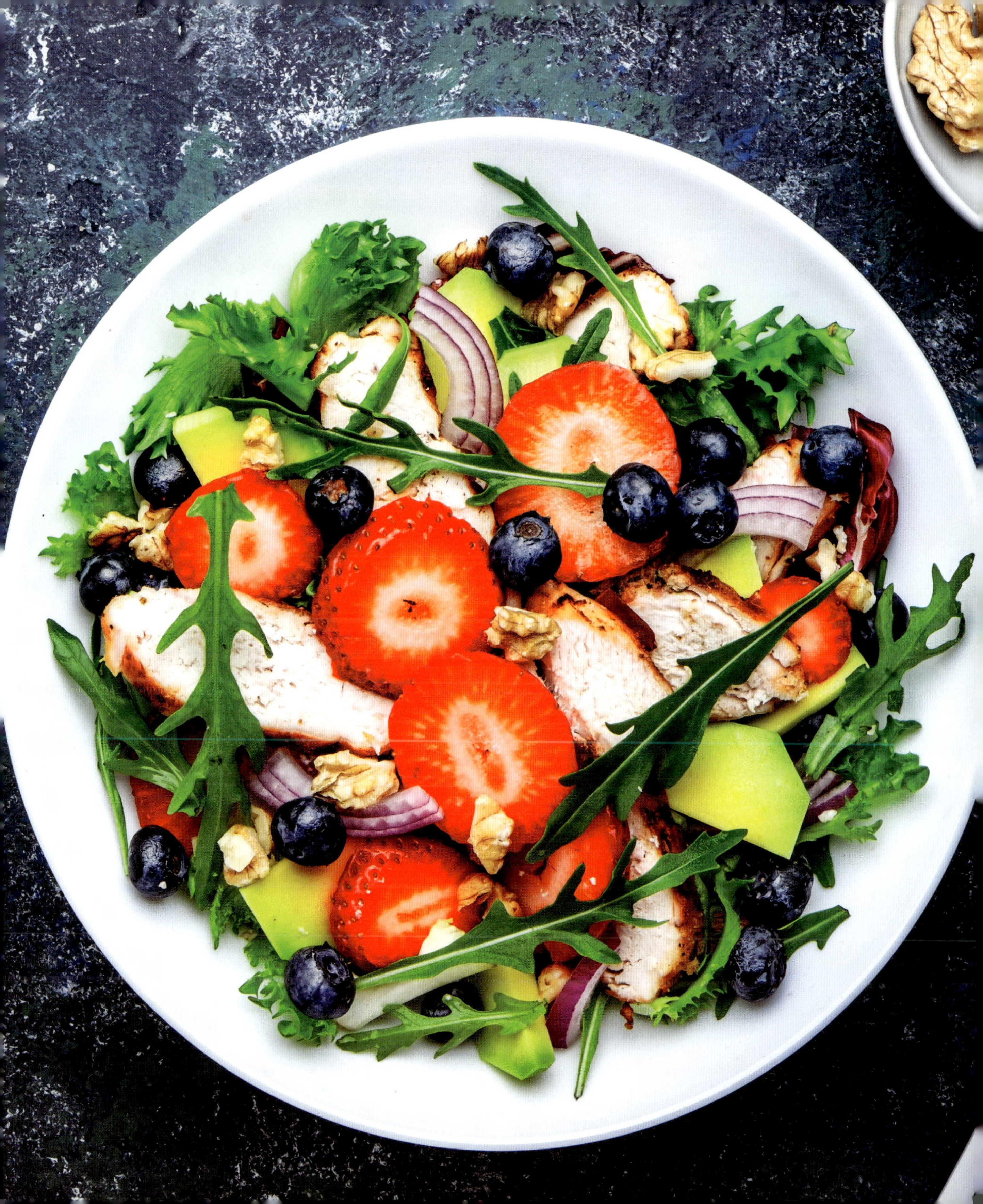

Mediterranean Tuna Salad

makes 4 servings

- ½ cup diced tomato
- 1 tablespoon olive oil
- 1 tablespoon lemon juice
- 2 teaspoons Dijon mustard
- ½ teaspoon garlic powder
- ¼ teaspoon salt
- ¼ teaspoon dried basil
- 2 cans (6 ounces each) solid white tuna packed in water, drained and flaked
- ½ cup diced celery
- ⅓ cup chopped fresh basil
- Red leaf lettuce leaves
- ½ pound steamed green beans
- 1 medium red bell pepper, seeded and cut into strips
- 8 cherry tomatoes, halved

1. Combine diced tomato, oil, lemon juice, mustard, garlic powder, salt and dried basil in large bowl; let stand 5 minutes.
2. Stir in tuna, celery and fresh basil. Cover and refrigerate 1 to 2 hours to allow flavors to blend, stirring once.
3. Line serving plates with lettuce leaves. Mound tuna salad in center; add green beans, bell pepper and cherry tomatoes to each plate.

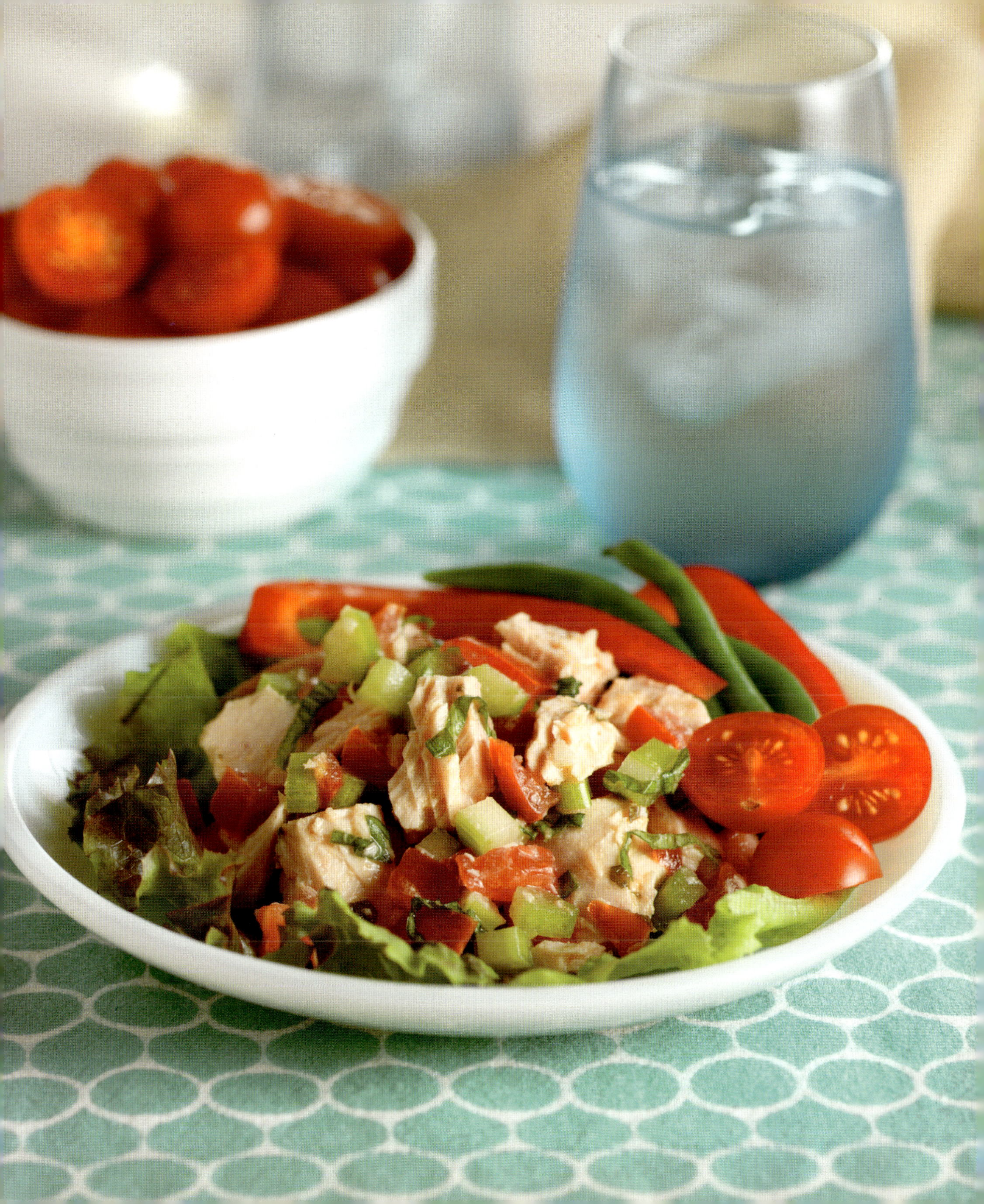

Cilantro-Stuffed Chicken Breasts

makes 4 servings

½ teaspoon garlic powder
1 cup packed fresh cilantro leaves
1 tablespoon plus 2 teaspoons soy sauce, divided
1 tablespoon olive oil
4 boneless chicken breasts with skin (about 5 ounces each)
1 tablespoon dark sesame oil

1. Preheat oven to 350°F. Line shallow baking pan with foil; top with wire rack.
2. Combine garlic powder and cilantro in food processor. Add 2 teaspoons soy sauce and olive oil; process until paste forms.
3. With rubber spatula or fingers, spread about 1 tablespoon cilantro mixture evenly under skin of each chicken breast, taking care not to puncture skin.
4. Place chicken on rack in prepared pan. Combine remaining 1 tablespoon soy sauce and sesame oil in small bowl. Brush half of mixture evenly over chicken.
5. Bake 25 minutes. Brush with remaining soy sauce mixture; bake 10 minutes or until no longer pink in center.

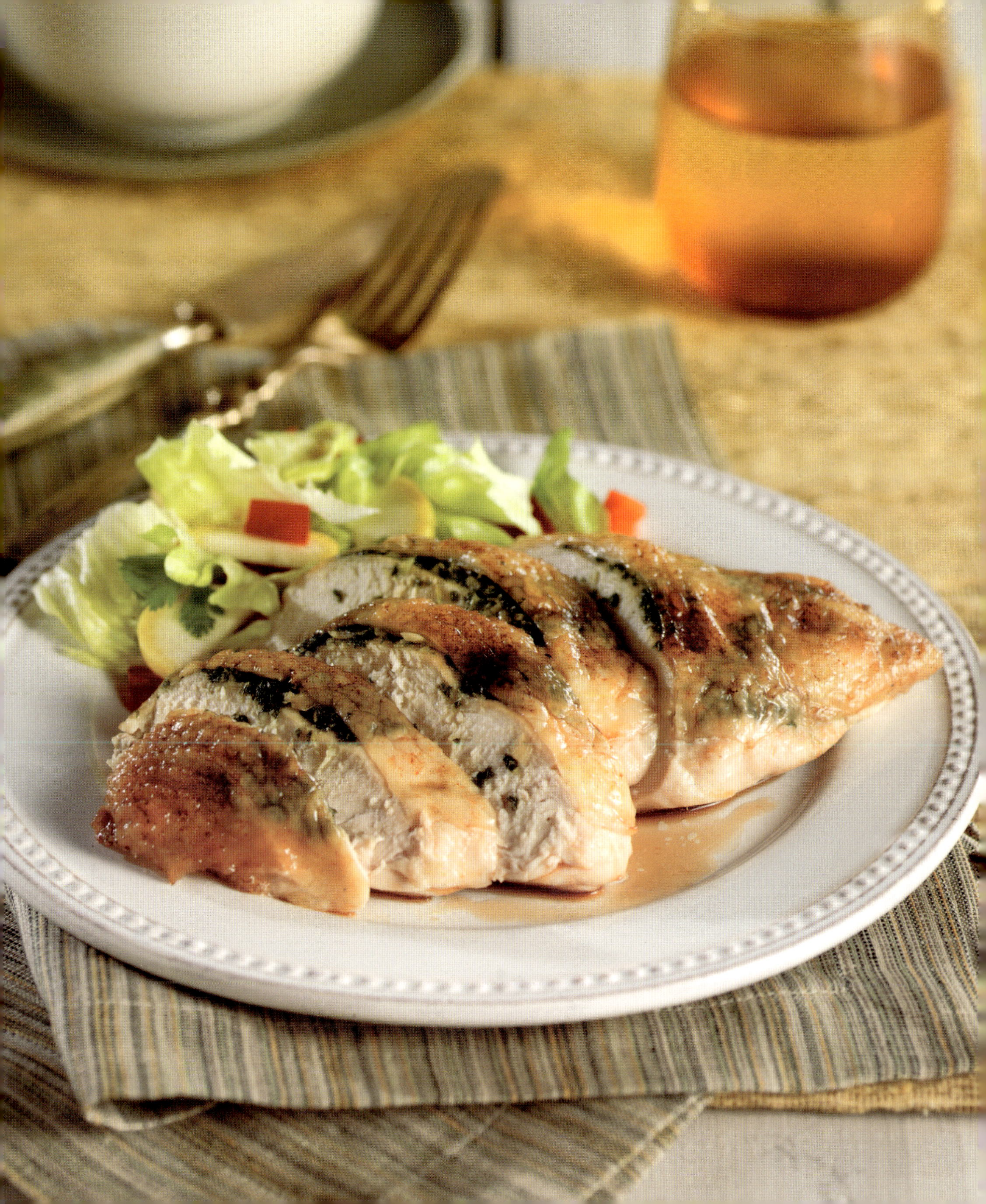

Crab Spinach Salad with Tarragon Dressing

makes 4 servings

- 12 ounces coarsely flaked cooked crabmeat *or* 2 packages (6 ounces each) frozen crabmeat, thawed and drained
- ½ cup chopped tomatoes
- 1 cup sliced cucumber
- 2 tablespoons sliced red onion
- ¼ cup fat-free salad dressing
- ¼ cup plain nonfat Greek yogurt
- ¼ cup chopped fresh parsley
- 2 tablespoons fat-free (skim) milk
- 2 teaspoons chopped fresh tarragon *or* ½ teaspoon dried tarragon
- ½ teaspoon garlic powder
- ¼ teaspoon hot pepper sauce
- 8 cups fresh spinach

1. Combine crabmeat, tomatoes, cucumber and onion in medium bowl.
2. Combine salad dressing, yogurt, parsley, milk, tarragon, garlic powder and hot pepper sauce in small bowl; mix well.
3. Line four salad plates with spinach. Spoon crabmeat mixture over spinach; drizzle with dressing.

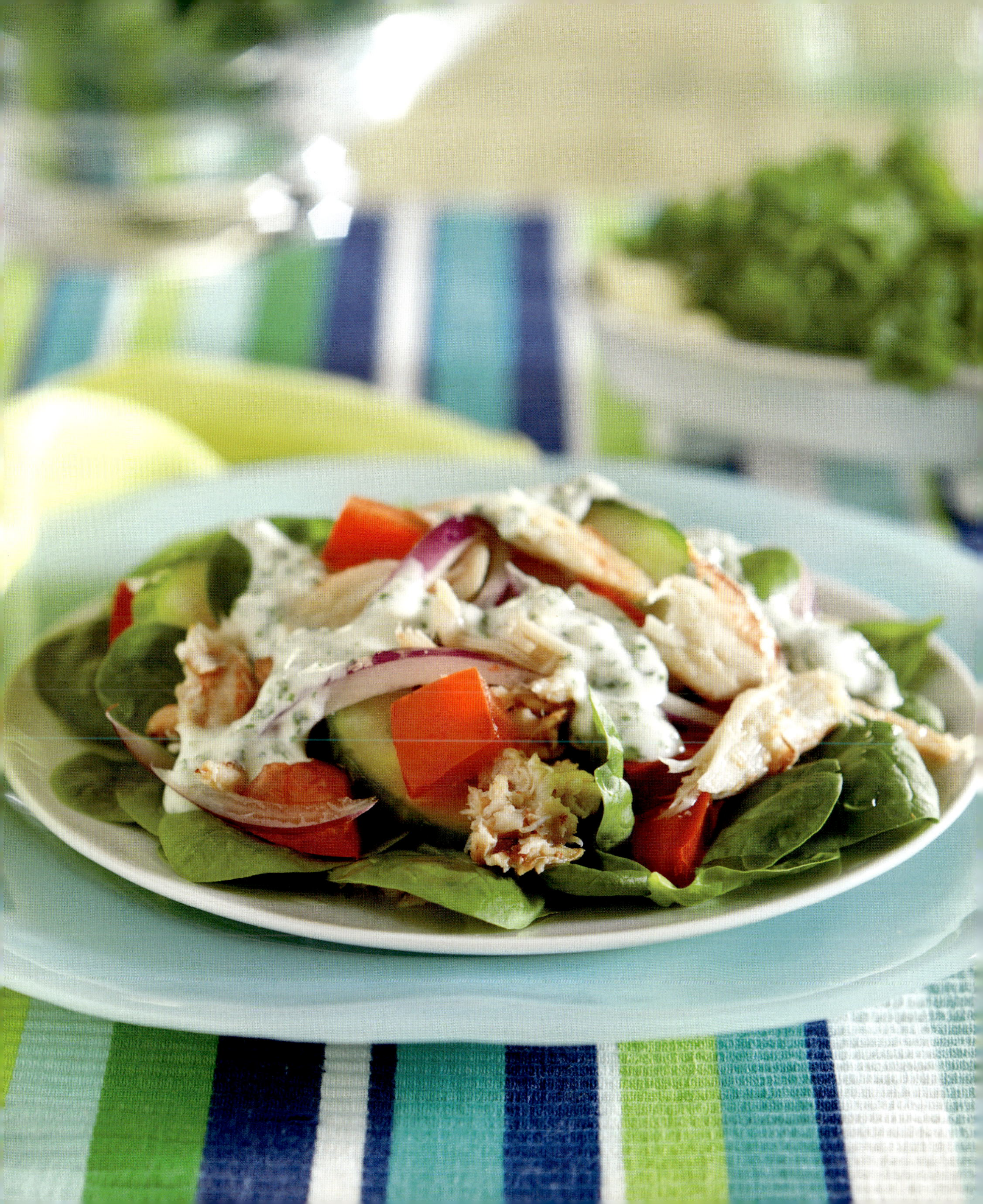

Thai Grilled Beef Salad

makes 4 servings

- **3 tablespoons Thai seasoning, divided**
- **1 beef flank steak (about 1 pound)**
- **2 tablespoons chopped fresh cilantro**
- **2 tablespoons chopped fresh basil**
- **1 red jalapeño pepper,* seeded and sliced into thin slivers *or* 2 red Thai peppers**
- **1 tablespoon finely chopped lemongrass**
- **Juice of 1 lime**
- **1 tablespoon fish sauce**
- **1 large carrot, grated**
- **1 cucumber, chopped**
- **4 cups assorted salad greens**

****Jalapeño peppers and Thai chili peppers and can sting and irritate the skin, so wear rubber gloves when handling peppers and do not touch your eyes.***

1. Prepare grill for direct grilling.
2. Sprinkle 1 tablespoon Thai seasoning over beef; turn to coat. Cover and let stand 15 minutes.
3. Grill steak, uncovered, over medium heat 17 to 21 minutes for medium rare (130° to 135°F) or to desired doneness, turning once. Transfer steak to cutting board; tent with foil and let stand 10 minutes.
4. Meanwhile, combine remaining 2 tablespoons Thai seasoning, cilantro, basil, jalapeño pepper, lemongrass, lime juice and fish sauce in medium bowl; mix well.
5. Cut steak into thin slices across the grain. Add steak, carrot and cucumber to dressing; toss to coat. Serve over salad greens.

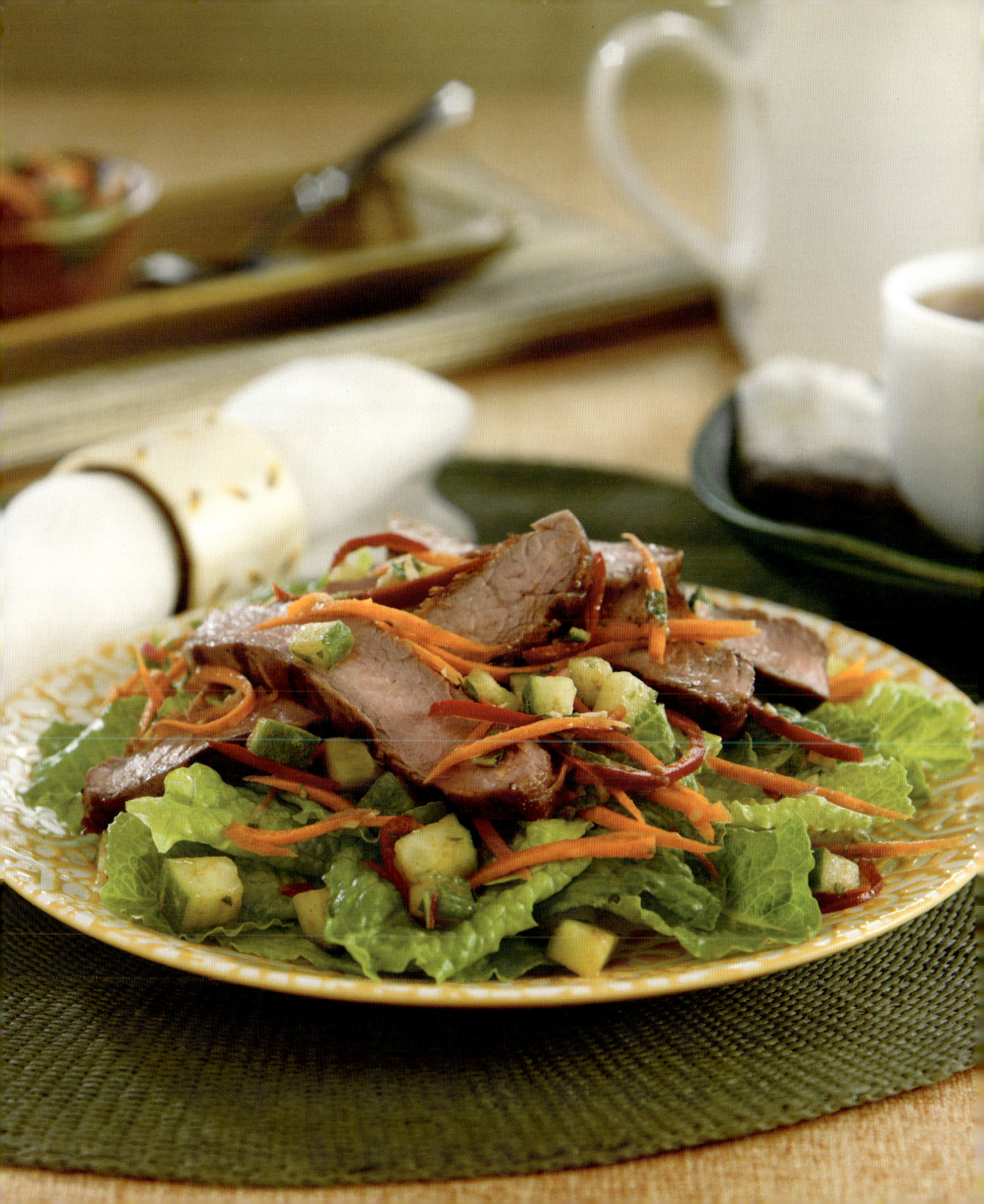

Chicken Kabobs over Quinoa

makes 4 servings

½ cup uncooked quinoa
1 cup water
1 jalapeño pepper,* seeded and finely chopped (optional)
3 teaspoons grated lemon peel, divided
½ teaspoon salt, divided
1 pound skinless boneless chicken breasts, cut into cubes
2 teaspoons chicken seasoning blend
4 asparagus spears, trimmed and sliced
8 grape tomatoes
4 green onions, cut into 3-inch pieces
2 tablespoons lemon juice
2 tablespoons extra virgin olive oil
¼ cup chopped fresh cilantro

**Jalapeño peppers can sting and irritate the skin, so wear rubber gloves when handling peppers and do not touch your eyes.*

1. Place quinoa in fine-mesh strainer; rinse well under cold running water. Bring 1 cup water to a boil in small saucepan; stir in quinoa. Reduce heat to low; cover and simmer 10 to 15 minutes or until quinoa is tender and water is absorbed. Remove from heat. Stir in jalapeño pepper, if desired, 2 teaspoons lemon peel and ¼ teaspoon salt. Keep warm.
2. Meanwhile, soak eight 12-inch wooden skewers in cold water 10 to 20 minutes. Sprinkle chicken cubes with seasoning blend. Thread asparagus, chicken, tomatoes and green onions onto skewers.
3. Combine lemon juice, remaining 1 teaspoon lemon peel, oil and remaining ¼ teaspoon salt in small bowl. Reserve half of mixture; brush remaining mixture over chicken and vegetable kabobs.
4. Oil grid. Prepare grill for direct cooking. Grill skewers 3 to 4 minutes on each side or until chicken is cooked through.
5. Brush skewers with reserved lemon juice mixture. Stir cilantro into quinoa; serve with skewers.

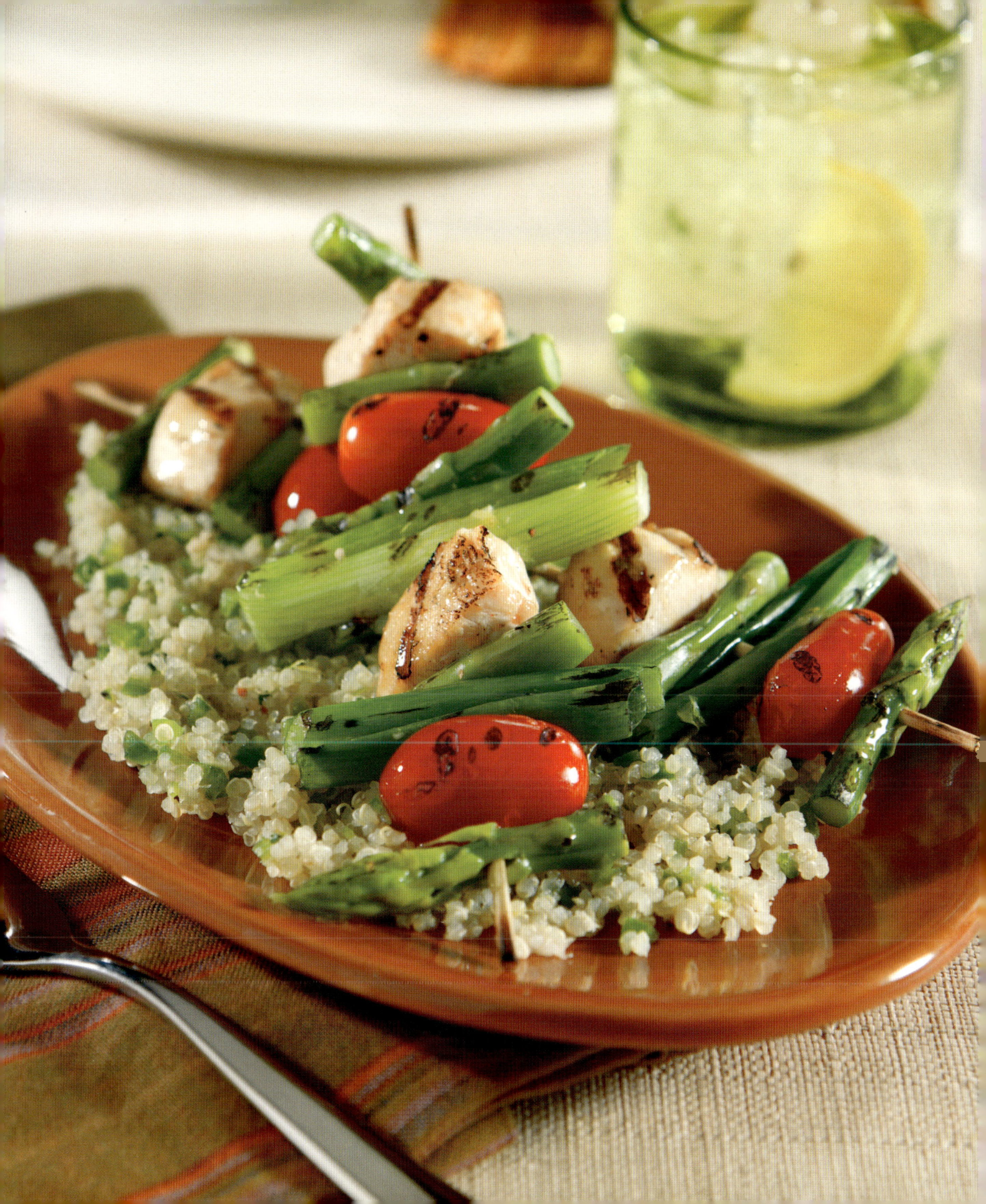

Spinach and Feta Farro Stuffed Peppers

makes 6 servings

- 1 tablespoon olive oil
- 1 package (5 ounces) baby spinach
- ½ cup sliced green onions
- 1 tablespoon chopped fresh oregano
- 1 package (8.8 ounces) quick-cooking farro, prepared according to package directions using vegetable broth in place of water
- ½ cup diced tomatoes
- ⅛ teaspoon black pepper
- 1 container (4 ounces) crumbled feta cheese, divided
- 3 large bell peppers, halved lengthwise, cores and ribs removed

1. Preheat oven to 350°F.
2. Heat oil in large skillet over medium-high heat. Add spinach, green onions and oregano; cook and stir 3 minutes. Stir in farro, tomatoes, black pepper and ½ cup cheese.
3. Spoon farro mixture into bell pepper halves (about ¾ cup each); place in shallow baking pan. Pour ¼ cup water into bottom of pan; cover with foil.
4. Bake 30 minutes or until bell peppers are crisp-tender and filling is heated through. Sprinkle with remaining cheese.

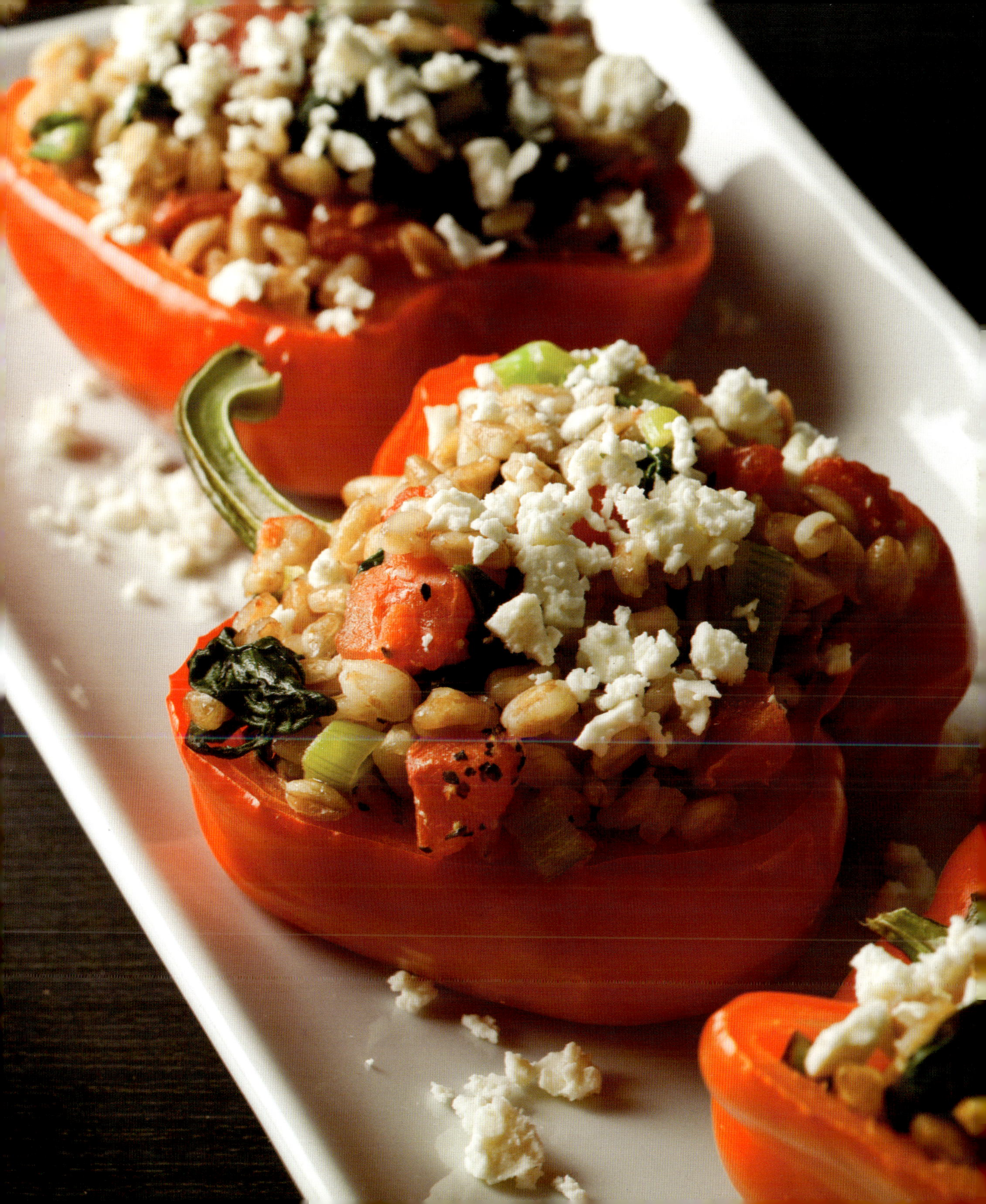

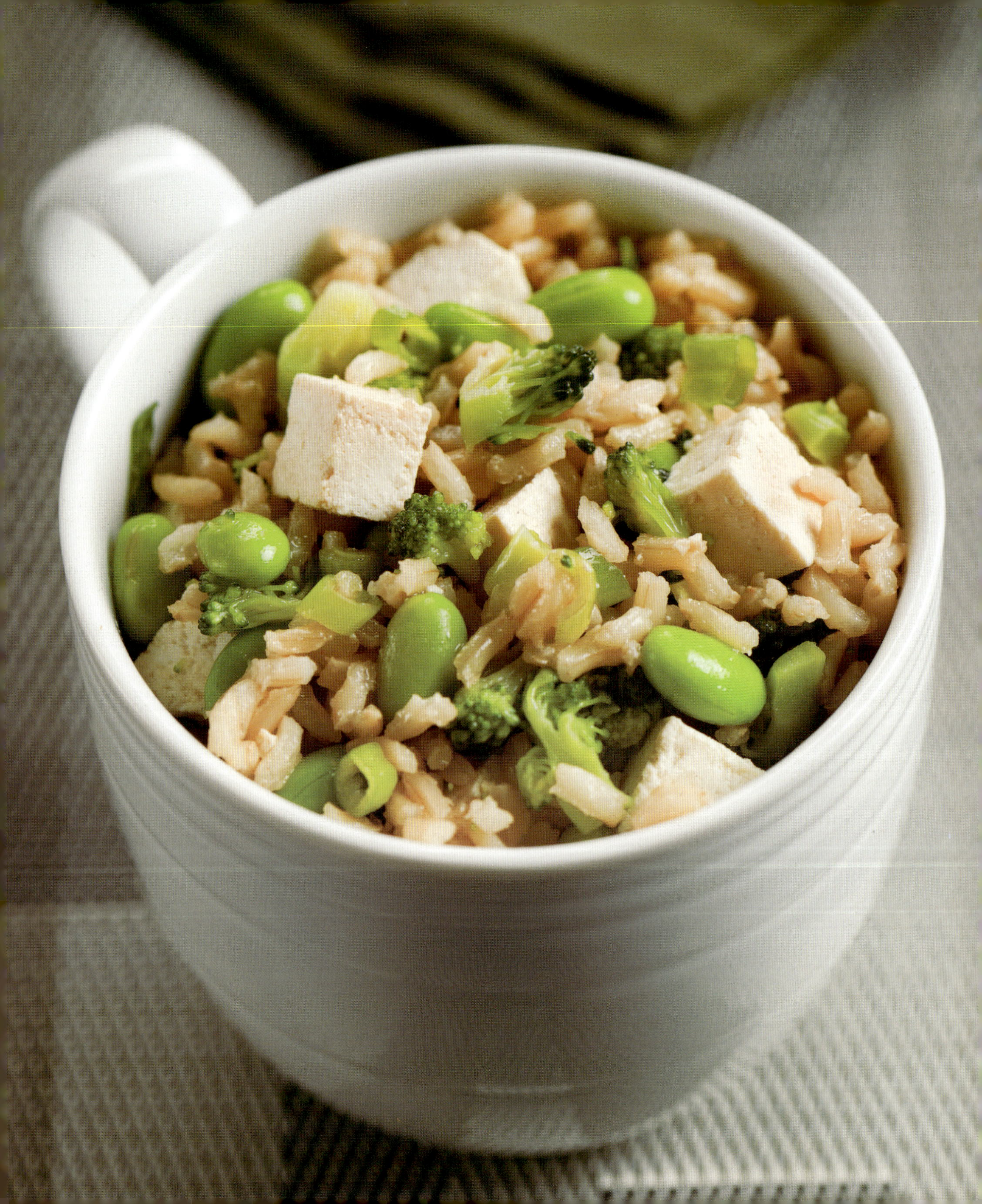

SOUPS & SIDES

Tofu "Fried" Rice

makes 1 serving

- **2 ounces extra firm tofu**
- **¼ cup finely chopped broccoli**
- **¼ cup thawed frozen shelled edamame**
- **⅓ cup cooked brown rice**
- **1 tablespoon chopped green onion**
- **½ teaspoon low-sodium soy sauce**
- **⅛ teaspoon garlic powder**
- **⅛ teaspoon sesame oil**

Microwave Directions

1. Press tofu between paper towels to remove excess water. Cut into ½-inch cubes.
2. Combine tofu, broccoli and edamame in large microwavable mug; mix well. Microwave on HIGH 1 minute.
3. Stir in rice, green onion, soy sauce, garlic powder and oil. Microwave 1 minute or until heated through. Stir well before serving.

Kale with Lemon and Garlic

makes 8 servings

- 2 bunches kale or Swiss chard (1 to 1¼ pounds)
- 1 tablespoon olive oil
- 1 clove garlic, minced
- ½ cup reduced-sodium chicken or vegetable broth
- ½ teaspoon salt (optional)
- ¼ teaspoon black pepper
- 1 lemon, cut into 8 wedges

1. Trim any tough stems from kale. Stack and thinly slice leaves. Heat oil in large saucepan over medium heat. Add garlic; cook 2 minutes, stirring frequently.
2. Stir in chopped kale and broth; cover and simmer 7 minutes. Stir kale; cover and simmer over medium-low heat 8 to 10 minutes or until kale is tender.
3. Stir in salt, if desired, and pepper. Squeeze wedge of lemon over each serving.

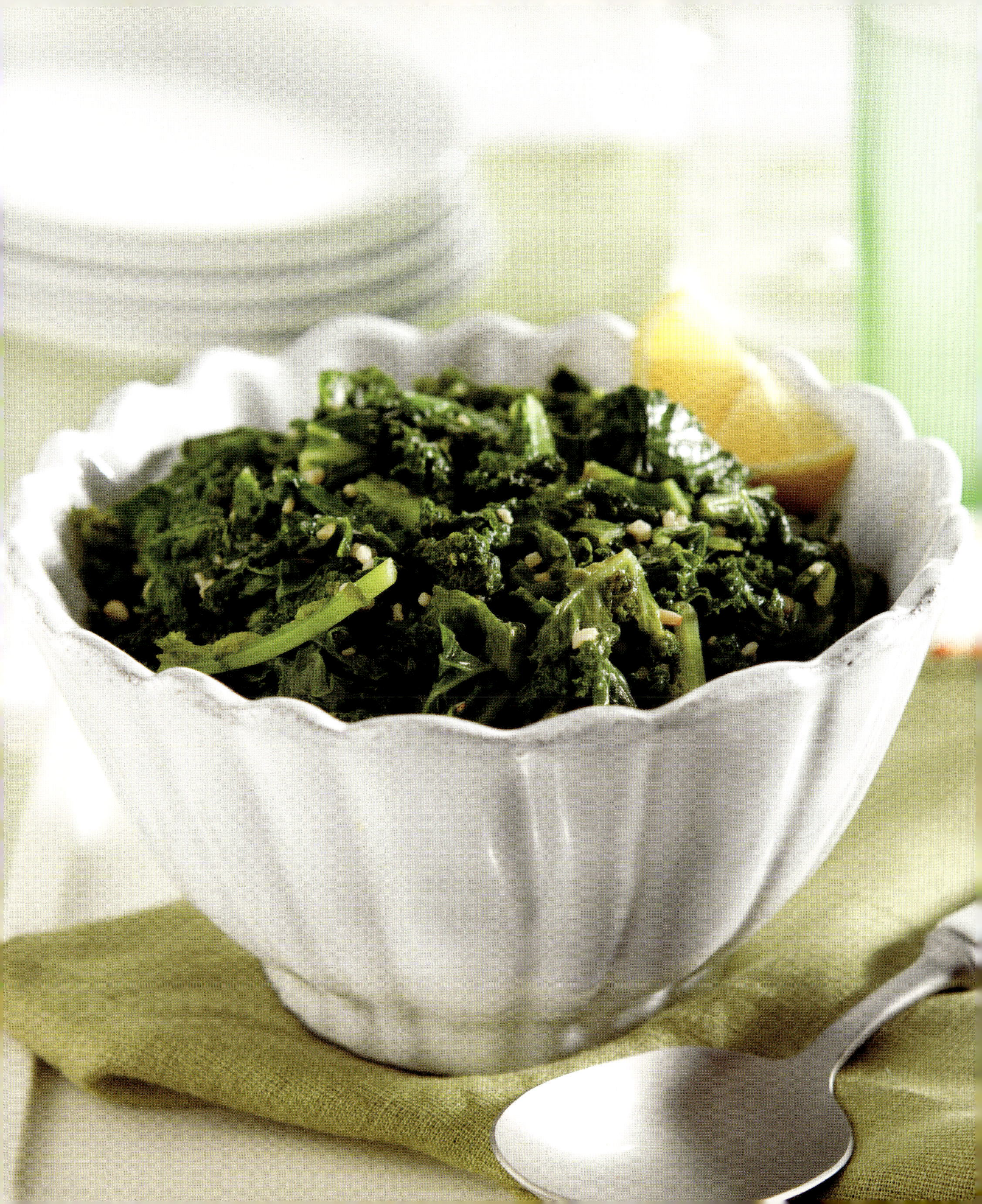

Wilted Spinach Salad with White Beans and Olives

makes 4 servings

- **1 tablespoon olive oil**
- **¼ cup chopped onion**
- **1 can (about 15 ounces) navy beans, rinsed and drained**
- **½ cup halved pitted kalamata or black olives**
- **1 package (9 ounces) baby spinach**
- **¾ cup cherry tomatoes, halved**
- **1½ tablespoons balsamic vinegar**
- **Black pepper (optional)**

1. Heat oil in large saucepan over medium heat. Add onion; cook 5 to 6 minutes or until onion is tender, stirring occasionally. Stir in beans and olives; cook until heated through.
2. Add spinach, tomatoes and vinegar; cover and cook 1 minute or until spinach is slightly wilted. Turn off heat; toss lightly. Transfer to serving plates; season with pepper, if desired.

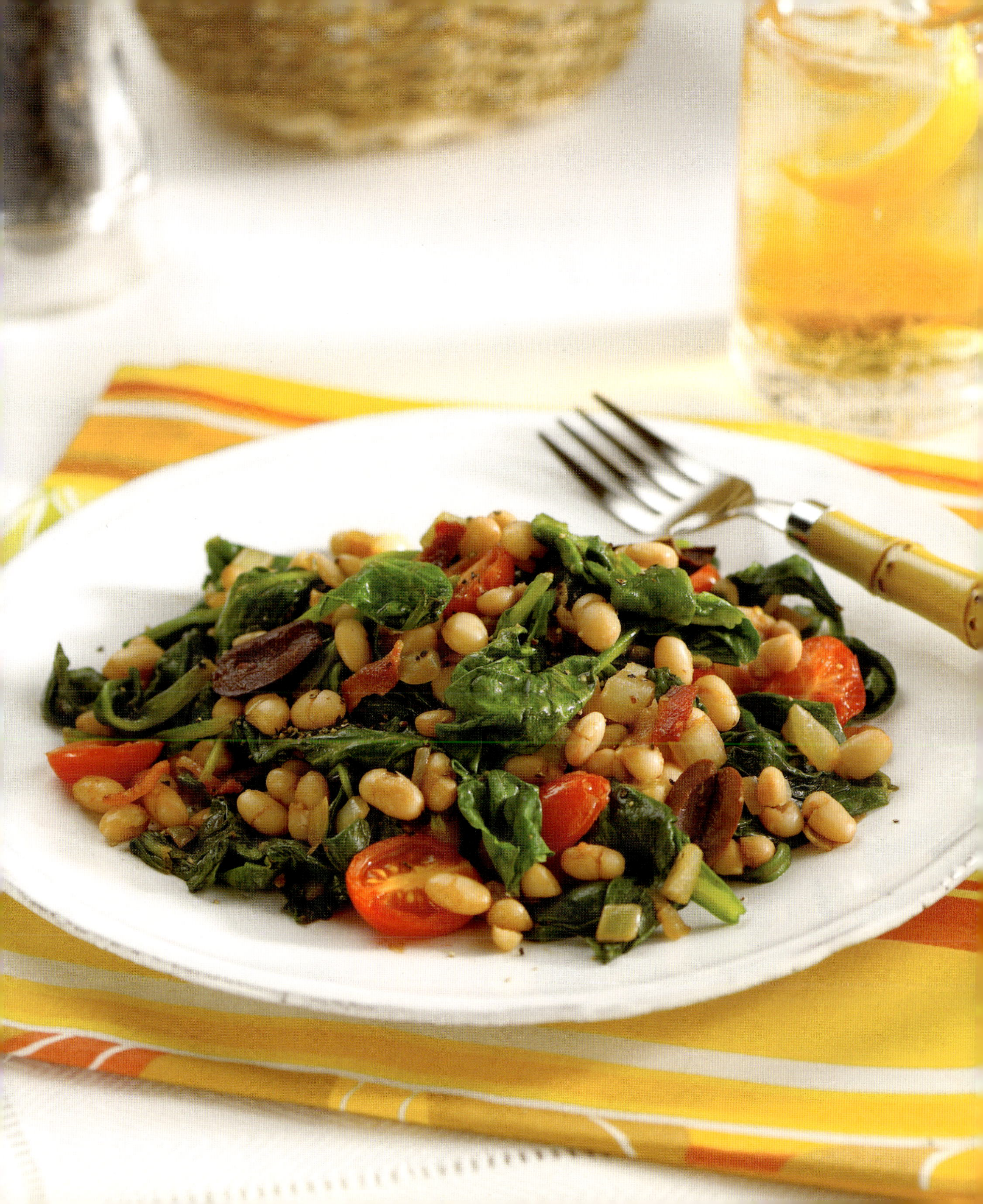

Chilled Cucumber Soup

makes 4 servings

- **1 large cucumber, peeled and coarsely chopped**
- **6 ounces plain nonfat Greek yogurt**
- **¼ cup packed fresh dill**
- **½ teaspoon salt (optional)**
- **⅛ teaspoon white pepper (optional)**
- **1½ cups fat-free reduced-sodium chicken or vegetable broth**
- **Sprigs fresh dill (optional)**

1. Place cucumber in food processor; process until finely chopped. Add yogurt, ¼ cup dill, salt and white pepper, if desired; process until smooth.
2. Transfer mixture to large bowl; stir in broth. Cover and refrigerate at least 2 hours or up to 24 hours. Garnish with dill sprigs.

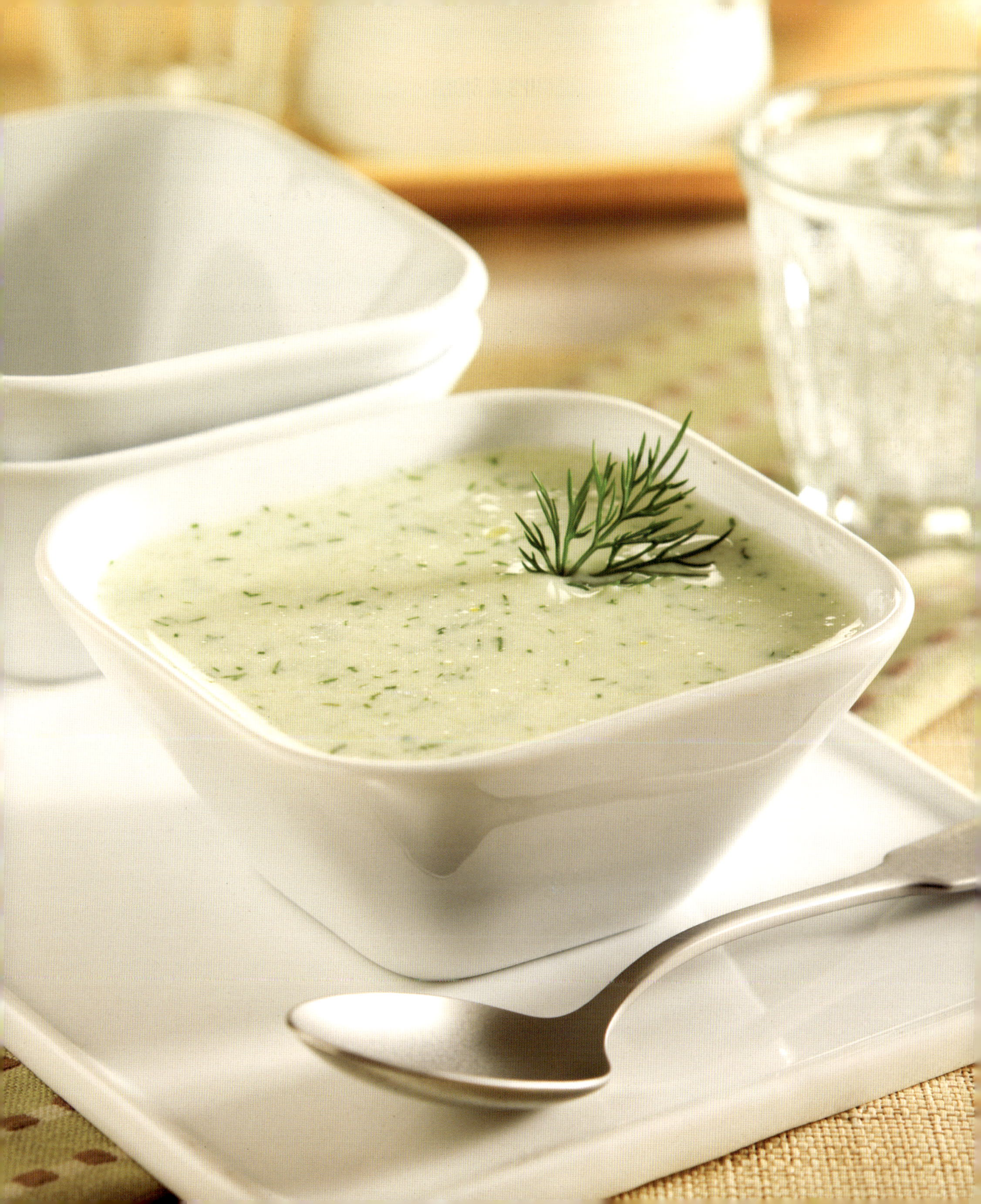

Acorn Squash Soup with Chicken and Red Pepper Meatballs

makes 2 servings

- 1 small to medium acorn squash (about ¾ pound)
- ½ pound ground lean chicken or turkey
- 1 red bell pepper, seeded and finely chopped
- 3 tablespoons cholesterol-free egg substitute
- 1 teaspoon dried parsley flakes
- 1 teaspoon ground coriander
- ½ teaspoon black pepper
- ¼ teaspoon ground cinnamon
- 3 cups reduced-sodium vegetable broth
- 2 tablespoons plain nonfat Greek yogurt (optional)
- Ground red pepper (optional)

1. Pierce squash skin with fork. Place in microwaveable dish; microwave on HIGH 8 to 10 minutes or until tender. Cool 10 minutes.
2. Meanwhile, combine chicken, bell pepper, egg substitute, parsley flakes, coriander, black pepper and cinnamon in large bowl, mix lightly. Shape mixture into eight meatballs.
3. Place meatballs in microwavable dish; microwave on HIGH 5 minutes or until cooked through. Set aside to cool.
4. Remove and discard seeds from cooled squash. Scrape squash flesh from shell into large saucepan; mash squash with potato masher. Add broth and meatballs to saucepan; cook over medium-high heat 12 minutes, stirring occasionally. Add additional liquid, if necessary.
5. Garnish each serving with 1 tablespoon yogurt and ground red pepper, if desired.

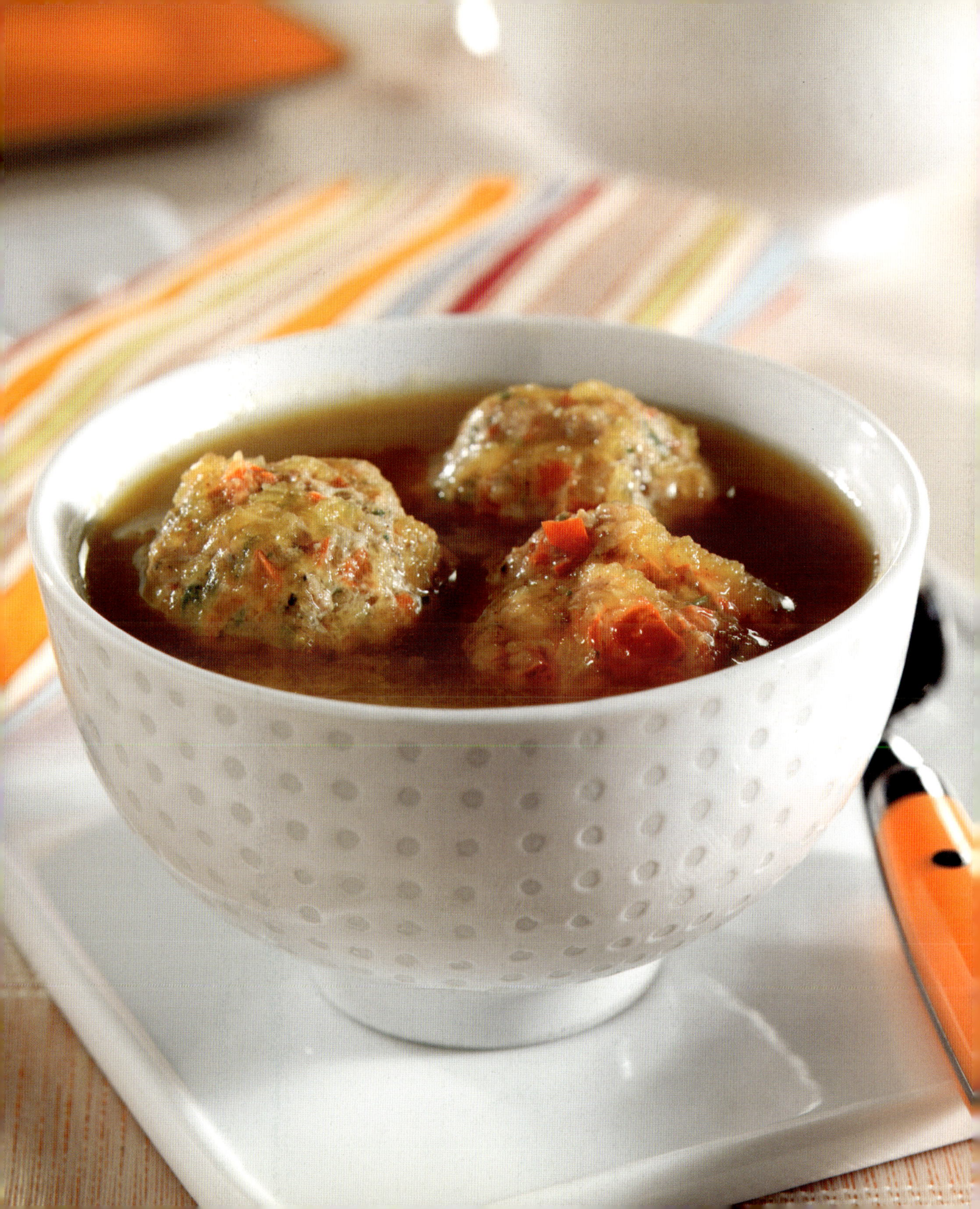

Mediterranean Stew

makes 6 servings

- 1 medium butternut or acorn squash, peeled and cut into 1-inch cubes
- 2 cups unpeeled eggplant, cut into 1-inch cubes
- 2 cups sliced zucchini
- 1 can (about 15 ounces) chickpeas, rinsed and drained
- 1 package (10 ounces) frozen cut okra
- 1 can (8 ounces) tomato sauce
- ¼ cup chopped onion
- 1 medium tomato, chopped
- 1 medium carrot, thinly sliced
- ½ cup reduced-sodium vegetable broth
- ¼ cup raisins
- ½ teaspoon ground cumin
- ½ teaspoon ground turmeric
- ¼ to ½ teaspoon ground red pepper
- ¼ teaspoon ground cinnamon
- ¼ teaspoon paprika
- 6 cups hot cooked couscous or brown rice
- Fresh chopped parsley (optional)

Slow Cooker Directions

1. Combine squash, eggplant, zucchini, chickpeas, okra, tomato sauce, onion, tomato, carrot, broth, raisins, cumin, turmeric, ground red pepper, cinnamon and paprika in slow cooker; mix well. Cover; cook on LOW 8 to 10 hours or until vegetables are crisp-tender.
2. Serve over couscous. Garnish with parsley.

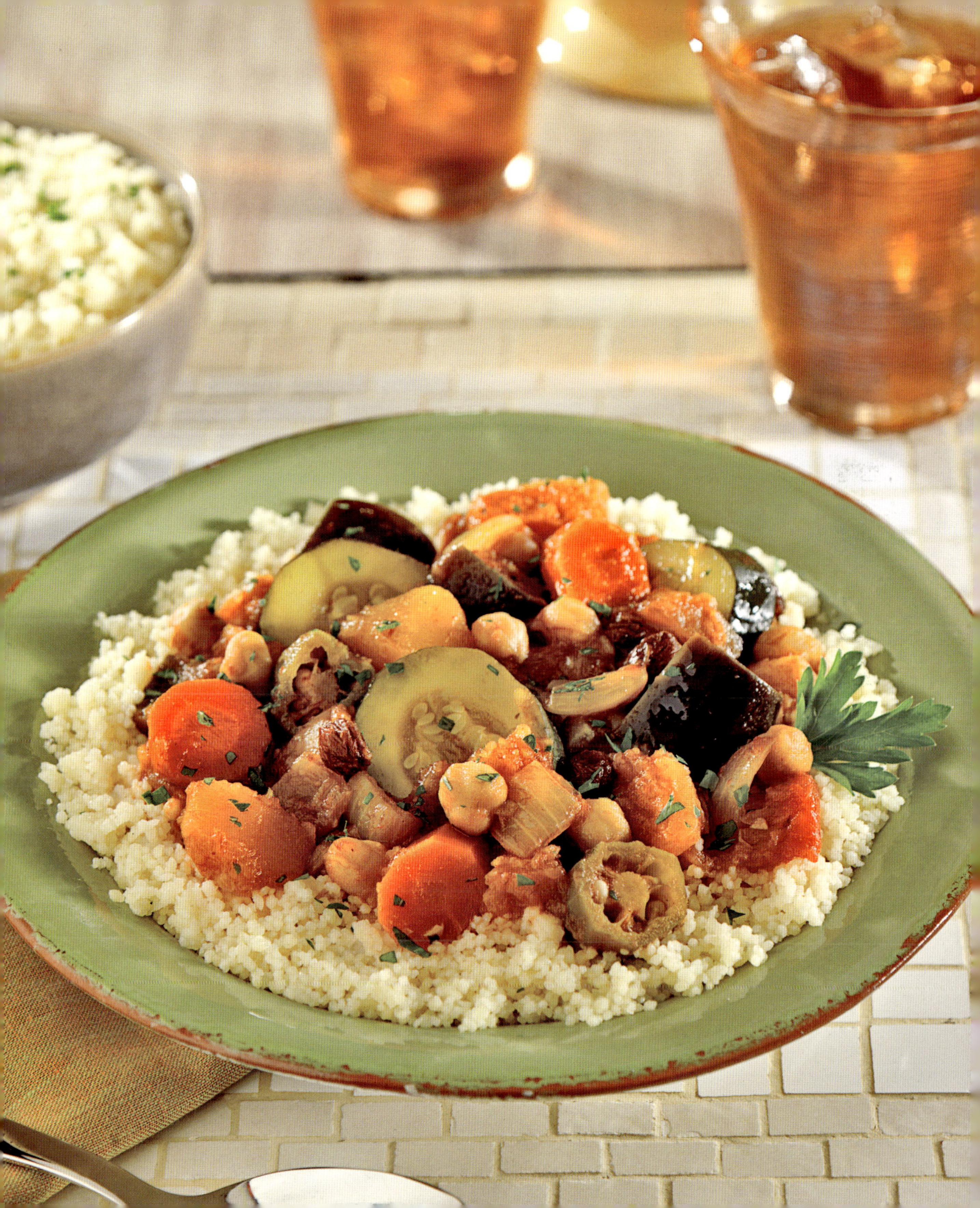

Couscous and Black Bean Salad

makes 4 servings

- **1⅓ cups cooked whole wheat couscous**
- **1 can (about 15 ounces) black beans, rinsed and drained**
- **½ cup cherry tomatoes**
- **2 tablespoons minced fresh chives or green onion**
- **1 tablespoon minced fresh cilantro**
- **1 small jalapeño pepper,* cored, seeded and minced (optional)**
- **2 teaspoons white wine vinegar**
- **1 teaspoon olive oil**
- **¼ teaspoon salt**
- **⅛ teaspoon black pepper**

****Jalapeño peppers can sting and irritate the skin, so wear rubber gloves when handling peppers and do not touch your eyes.***

1. Combine couscous and black beans in large bowl. Cut tomatoes in half lengthwise. Add tomatoes to couscous. Stir in chives, cilantro and jalapeño pepper, if desired; mix gently.
2. Whisk vinegar, oil, salt and black pepper in small bowl until well blended. Pour over salad; toss lightly to coat.

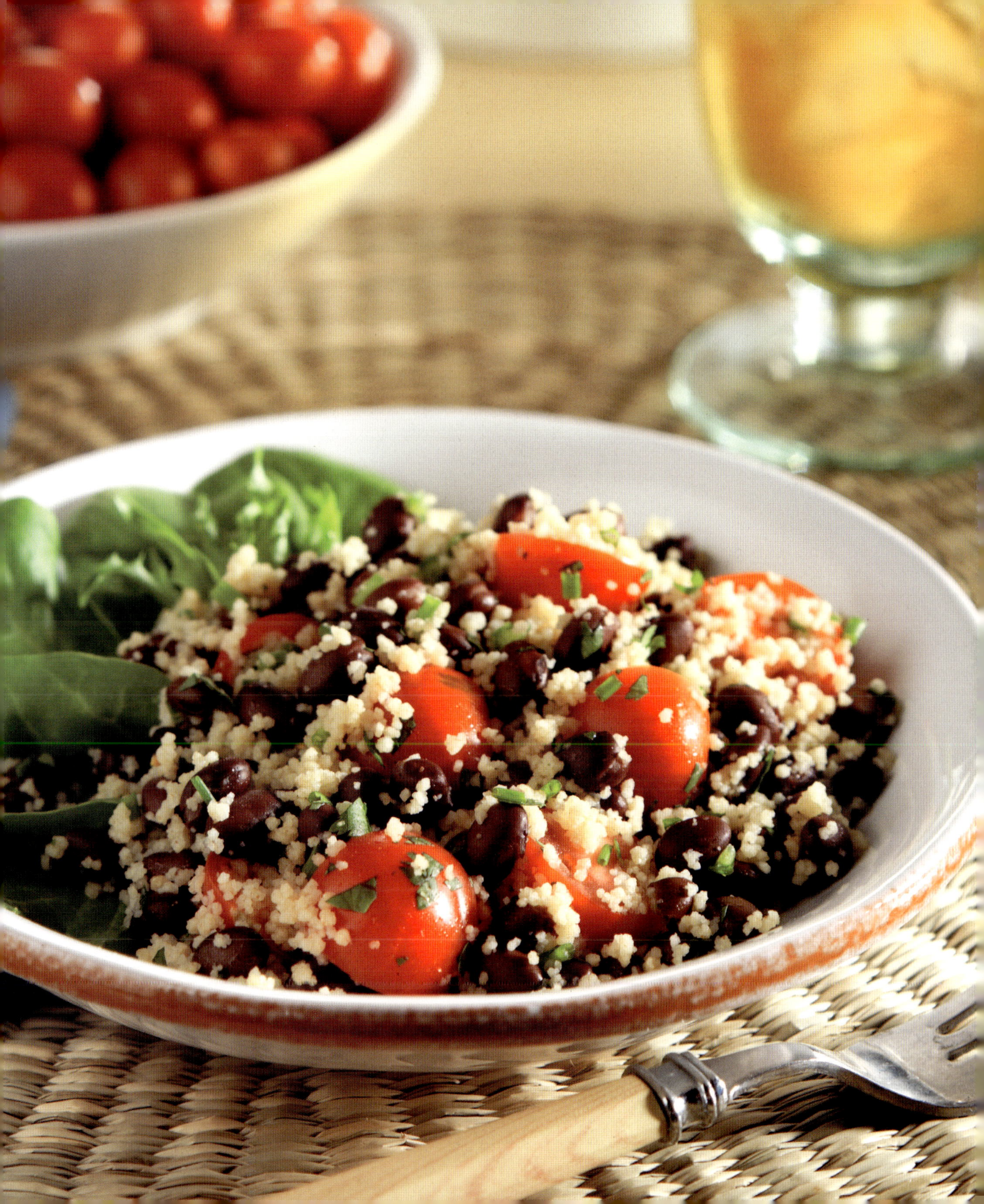

Cucumber-Jicama Salad

makes 6 servings

- 1 cucumber, unpeeled
- 1 jicama (1¼ to 1½ pounds)
- ¼ cup thinly slivered red onion (optional)
- 2 tablespoons lime juice
- ½ teaspoon grated lime peel
- ¼ teaspoon salt
- ⅛ teaspoon crumbled dried de árbol chile or red pepper flakes
- 3 tablespoons vegetable oil
- Leaf lettuce
- Lime wedges (optional)

1. Cut cucumber lengthwise in half; scoop out and discard seeds. Cut halves crosswise into ⅛-inch-thick slices. Peel jicama. Cut lengthwise into eight wedges; cut wedges crosswise into ⅛-inch-thick slices.
2. Combine cucumber, jicama and onion, if desired, in large bowl; stir gently.
3. Combine lime juice, lime peel, salt and chile in small bowl. Gradually add oil, whisking constantly, until dressing is well blended.
4. Pour dressing over salad; toss lightly to coat. Cover and refrigerate 1 to 2 hours to blend flavors.
5. Serve over lettuce; garnish with lime wedges.

TIP To add a decorative touch to cucumber slices, score the skin of a cucumber by pulling the tines of a dinner fork along the length of the cucumber. Rotate the cucumber and repeat until completely scored. Then cut the cucumber crosswise into slices.

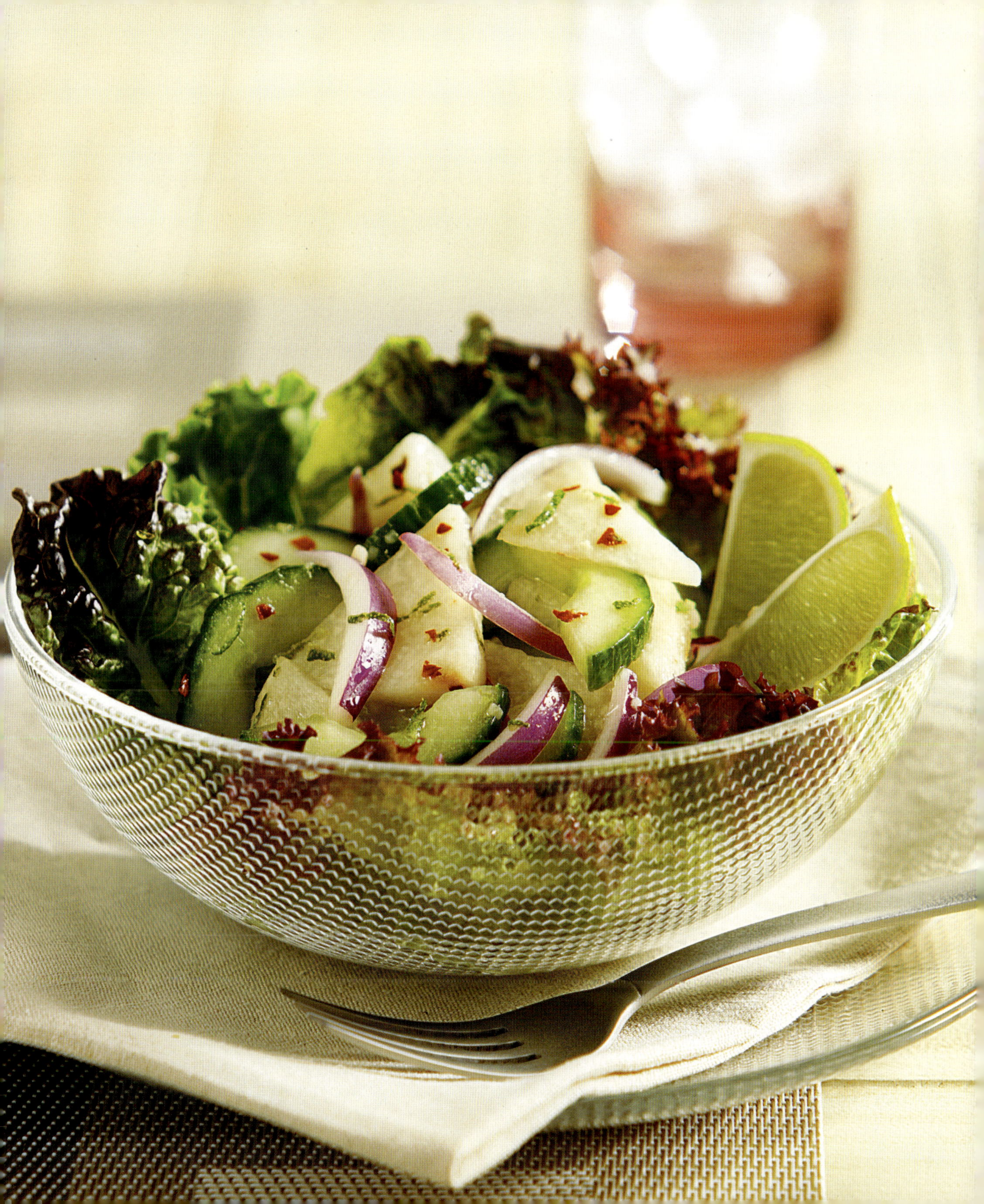

Spinach-Pine Nut Whole Grain Pilaf

makes 6 servings

- **2 cups hot cooked brown rice**
- **1½ ounces pine nuts or slivered almonds, toasted**
- **2 ounces spinach leaves, coarsely chopped**
- **1 tablespoon extra virgin olive oil**
- **1 teaspoon dried basil**
- **½ teaspoon salt**
- **¼ teaspoon red pepper flakes**

Place hot rice in large bowl; fluff with fork. Add pine nuts, spinach, oil, basil, salt and red pepper flakes; toss gently until spinach is slightly wilted.

TIP For this quick pilaf, you can use leftover brown rice, a package of ready-to-use cooked brown rice or cook the rice before preparing the pilaf. To cook brown rice, rinse 1 cup rice in a fine-mesh strainer under cold running water. Combine the rice with 2 cups water and ¼ teaspoon salt in a medium saucepan; bring to a boil over medium-high heat. Reduce the heat to low; cover and simmer about 30 minutes or until all the liquid is absorbed. Remove from the heat and let stand, covered, 10 minutes before fluffing the rice with a fork. One cup of uncooked rice yields about 3 cups of cooked rice; leftover rice can be stored in the refrigerator up to 5 days.

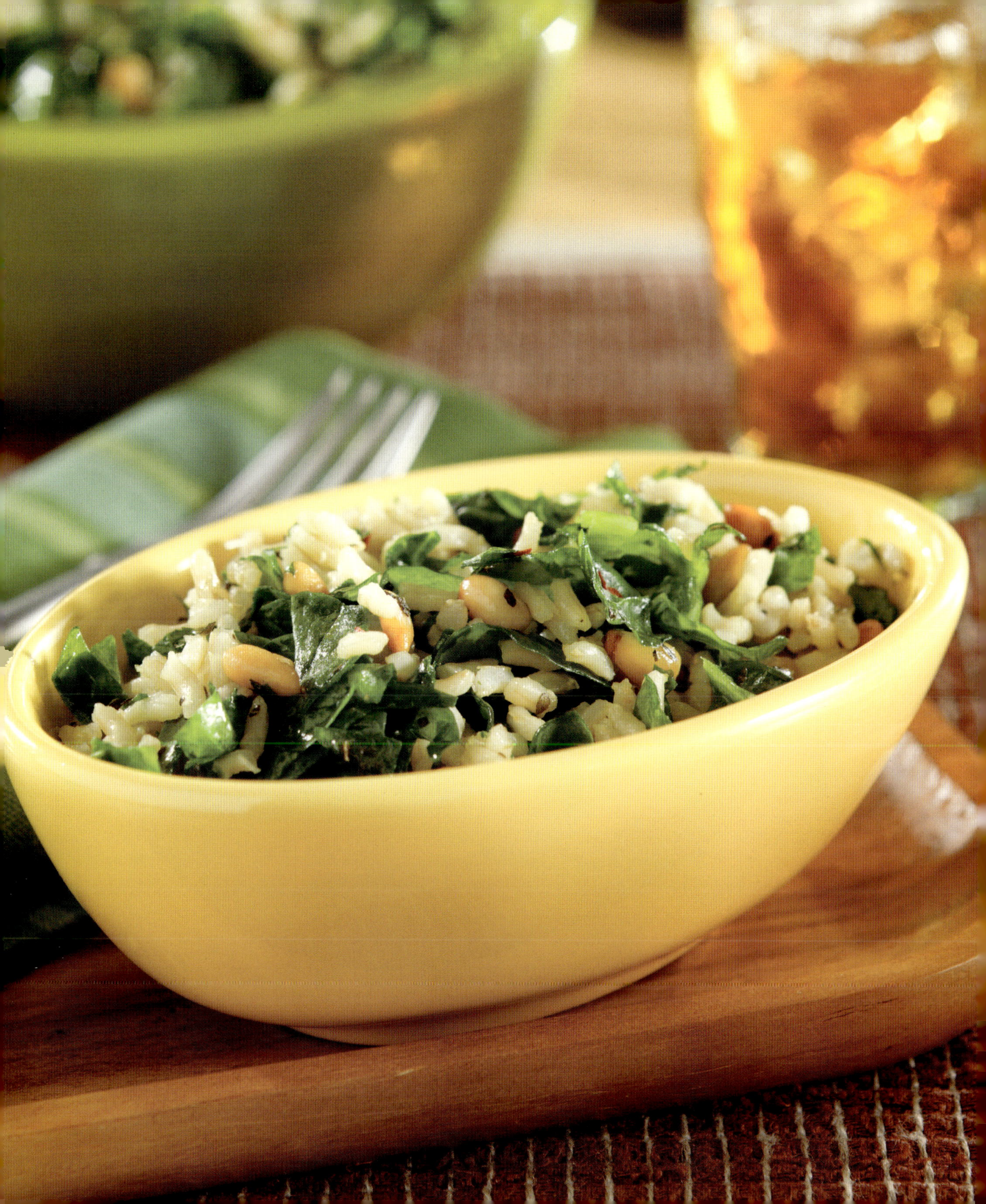

Favorite Green Beans

makes 6 servings

1 pound green beans
2 tablespoons olive oil
¼ cup grated Parmesan cheese
½ teaspoon garlic powder

1. Bring 1 quart of water to a boil in large saucepan. Add green beans and boil 3 minutes. Drain beans, shaking off any excess water.
2. Heat oil in large skillet over medium heat. Add green beans to skillet; cook 5 minutes, stirring occasionally.
3. Remove from heat; sprinkle with Parmesan cheese and garlic powder. Serve warm.

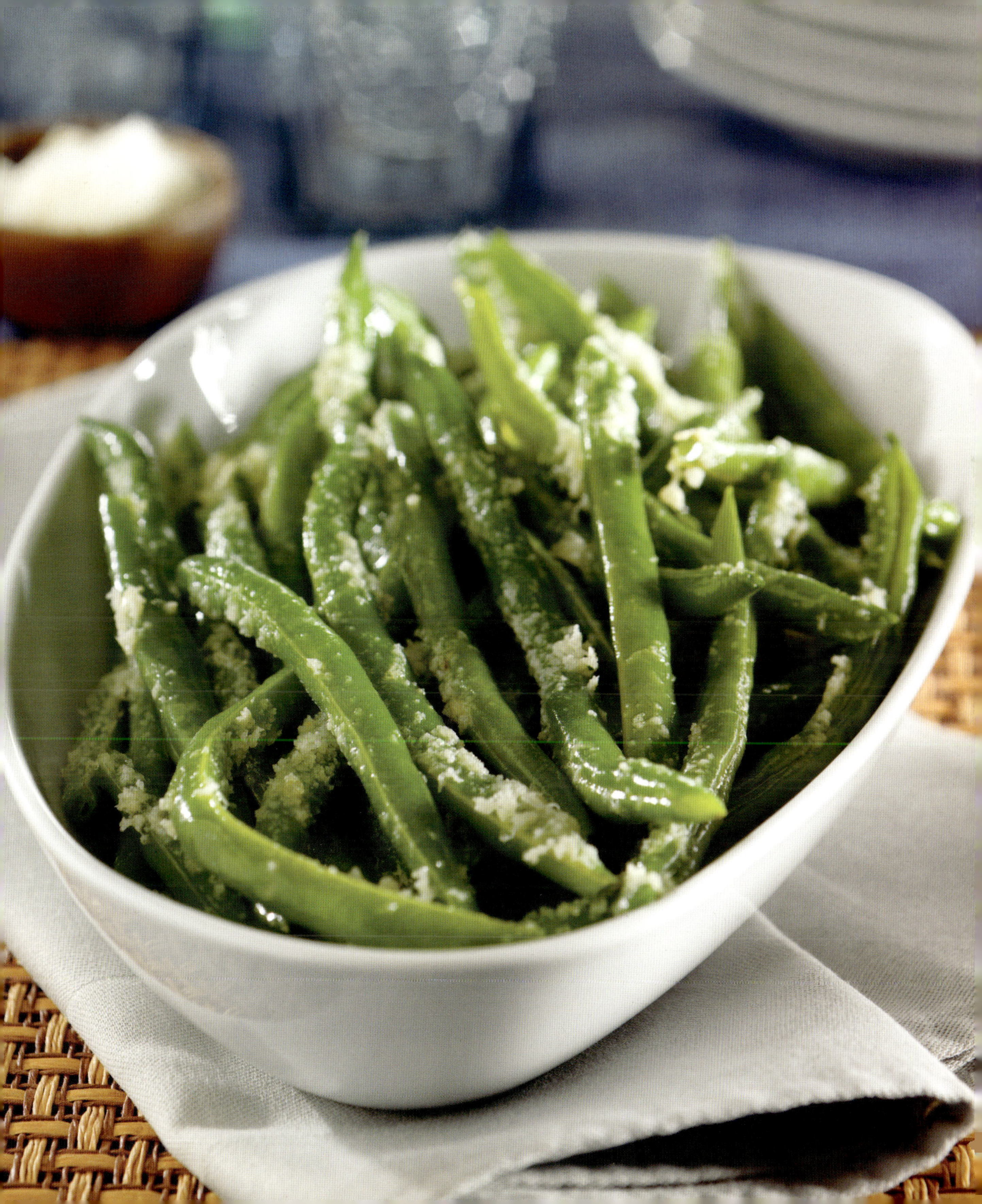

Mashed Sweet Potatoes and Parsnips

makes 6 servings

- 2 large sweet potatoes (about 1¼ pounds), peeled and cut into 1-inch pieces
- 2 medium parsnips (about ½ pound), peeled and cut into ½-inch slices
- ¼ cup unsweetened canned coconut milk
- 1 tablespoon butter
- ½ teaspoon salt
- ⅛ teaspoon ground nutmeg
- ¼ cup chopped fresh chives

1. Combine sweet potatoes and parsnips in large saucepan. Cover with cold water; bring to a boil over high heat. Reduce heat to low; simmer, uncovered, 15 minutes or until vegetables are tender.
2. Drain vegetables; return to saucepan. Add milk, butter, salt and nutmeg; mash with potato masher over low heat until desired consistency is reached. Stir in chives.

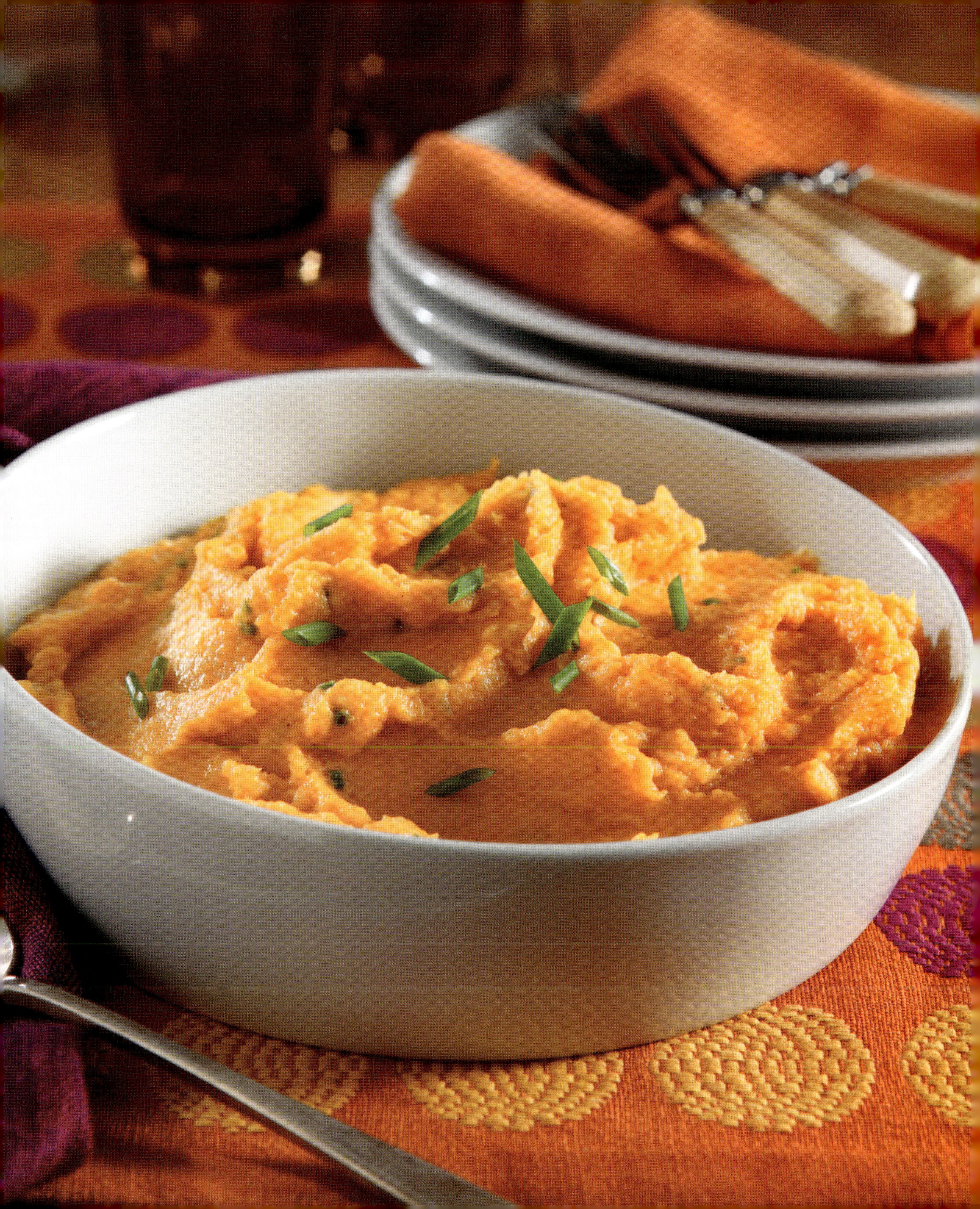

Pepper and Squash Gratin

makes 8 servings

1 unpeeled russet potato (12 ounces)
8 ounces yellow summer squash, thinly sliced
8 ounces zucchini, thinly sliced
2 cups frozen bell pepper stir-fry blend, thawed
1 teaspoon dried oregano
½ teaspoon salt
⅛ teaspoon black pepper (optional)
½ cup grated Parmesan cheese or shredded reduced-fat sharp Cheddar cheese (optional)
1 tablespoon olive oil

1. Preheat oven to 375°F. Spray 12×8-inch baking dish with nonstick cooking spray.
2. Pierce potato several times with fork. Microwave on HIGH 3 minutes. Cut potato into thin slices.
3. Layer half of potato slices, yellow squash, zucchini, bell pepper blend, oregano, salt, black pepper and cheese, if desired, in prepared baking dish. Repeat layers. Drizzle with oil. Cover tightly with foil.
4. Bake 25 minutes or just until vegetables are tender. Uncover; bake 10 minutes or until lightly browned.

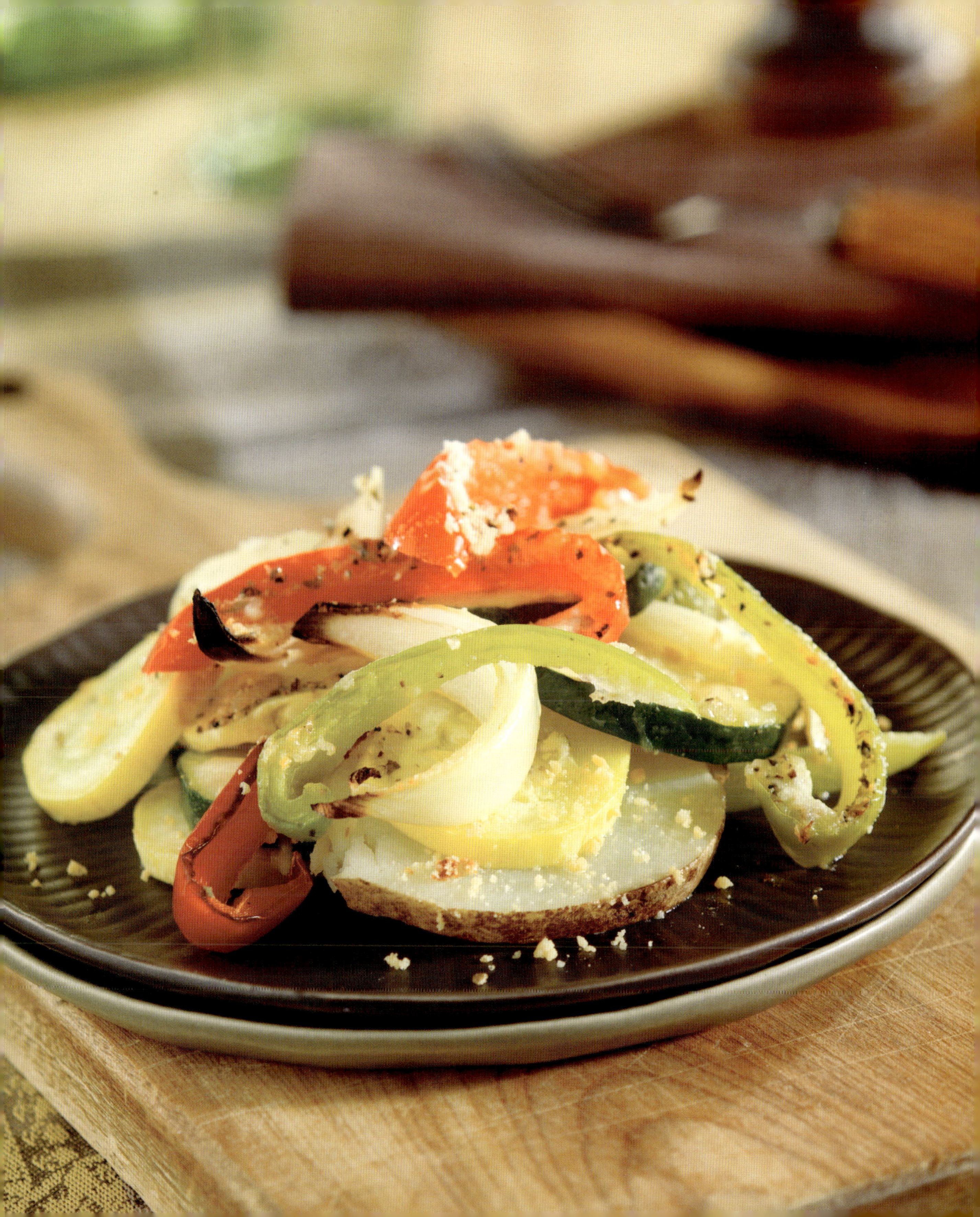

Heirloom Tomato Quinoa Salad

makes 4 servings

1 cup uncooked quinoa
2 cups water
2 tablespoons olive oil
1 tablespoon lemon juice
½ teaspoon garlic powder
½ teaspoon salt
1 cup assorted heirloom grape tomatoes (red, yellow or a combination), halved
¼ cup crumbled reduced-fat feta cheese (optional)
¼ cup chopped fresh basil, plus additional basil leaves for garnish

1. Place quinoa in fine-mesh strainer; rinse well under cold running water. Bring 2 cups water to a boil in small saucepan; stir in quinoa. Reduce heat to low; cover and simmer 10 to 15 minutes or until quinoa is tender and water is absorbed.
2. Meanwhile, whisk oil, lemon juice, garlic powder and salt in large bowl until well blended. Gently stir in tomatoes and quinoa. Cover and refrigerate at least 30 minutes.
3. Sprinkle with cheese, if desired, just before serving. Top each serving with 1 tablespoon chopped basil. Garnish with additional basil leaves.

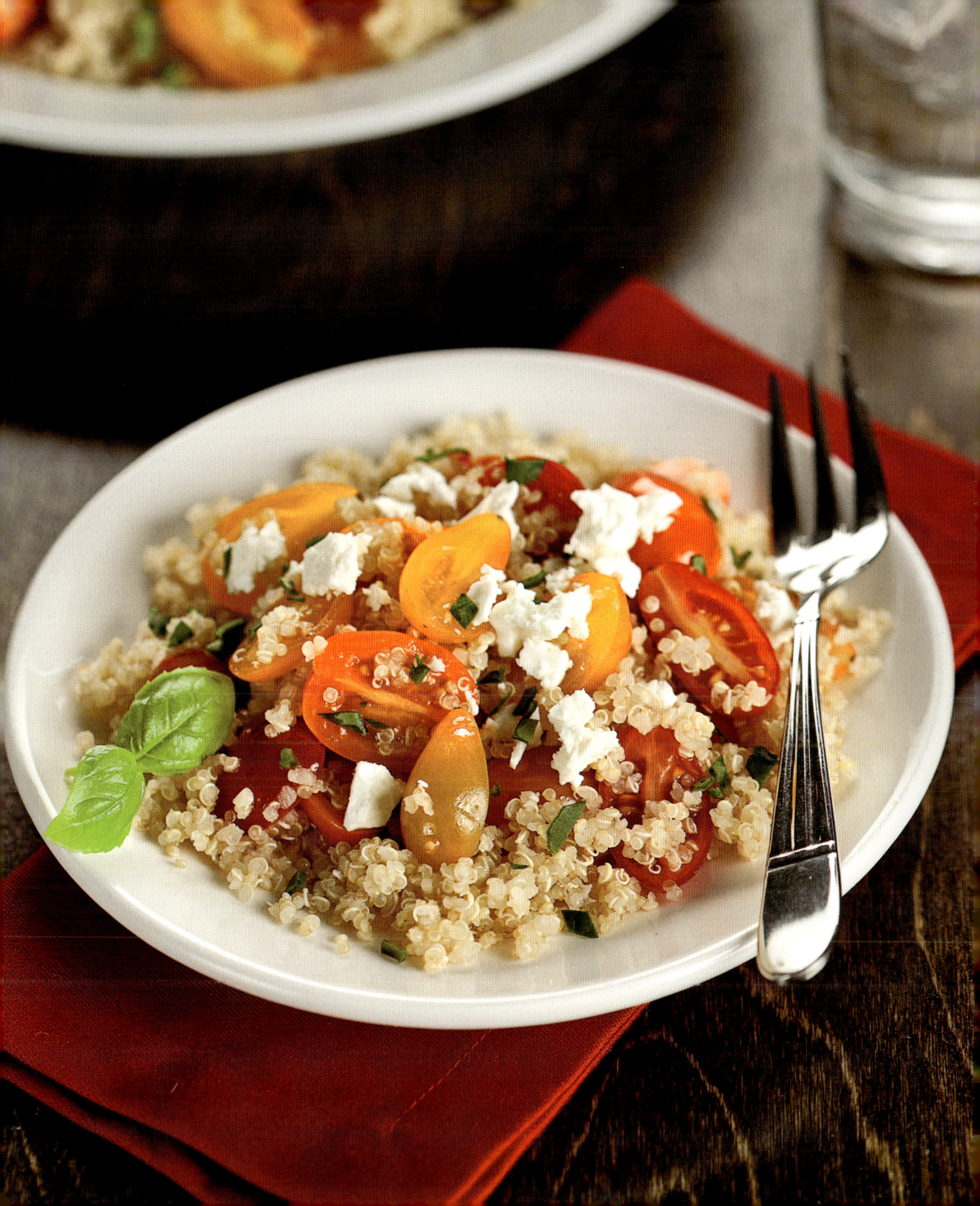

Tabbouleh-Style Amaranth Salad

makes 5 to 6 servings

- **2½ cups water**
- **¾ cup dried amaranth***
- **2 cups chopped fresh parsley**
- **½ cup grape tomatoes, quartered**
- **¼ cup diced red onion**
- **1 ounce (¼ cup) pine nuts, toasted**
- **3 tablespoons capers, drained (optional)**
- **2 tablespoons cider vinegar or red wine vinegar**
- **1 tablespoon extra virgin olive oil**
- **½ teaspoon garlic powder**
- **¼ teaspoon salt**
- **⅛ teaspoon red pepper flakes (optional)**
- **¾ cup (4 ounces) reduced-fat feta cheese, crumbled**

Amaranth is an ancient whole grain that is very high in protein and fiber. In addition, it's gluten-free and a good source of iron and vitamin C. You can find it at the supermarket with the other grains or in bulk bins at health food stores.

1. Combine water and amaranth in large saucepan; bring to a boil over high heat. Reduce heat, cover and simmer 20 minutes or until most of water is absorbed. (It will have a very soft consistency.)
2. Meanwhile, combine parsley, tomatoes, onion, pine nuts, capers, if desired, vinegar, oil, garlic powder, salt and red pepper flakes in medium bowl; set aside.
3. Place amaranth in fine-mesh strainer; rinse well under cold running water until completely cooled. Shake off excess liquid.
4. Add amaranth to parsley mixture; mix well. Stir in feta; toss gently to blend.

TIP It's important that the amaranth is drained in a fine-mesh strainer. The grain is very small and will slip through a traditional strainer.

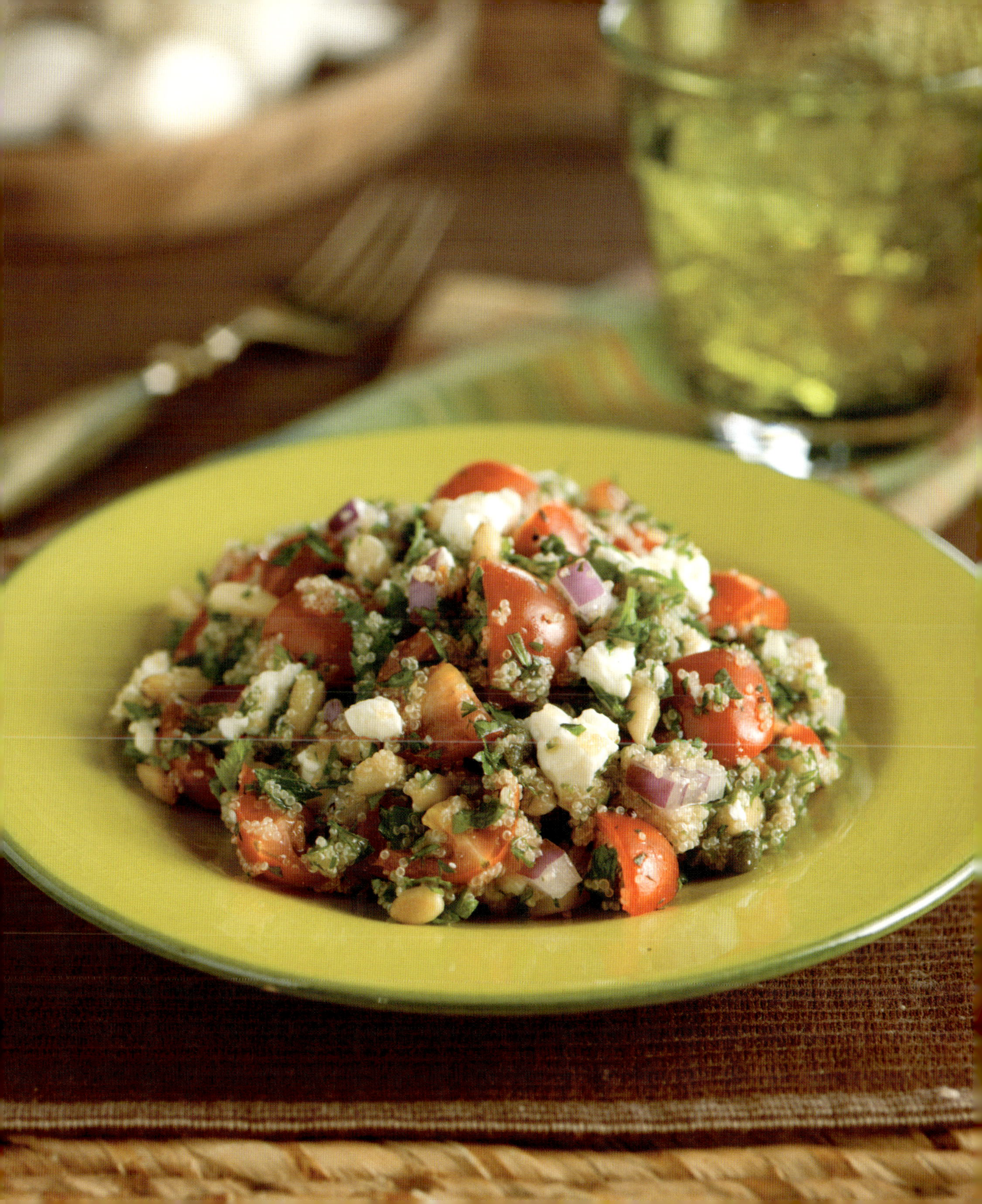

Roman Spinach Soup

makes 8 servings

- 6 cups fat-free reduced-sodium chicken broth
- 1 cup cholesterol-free egg substitute
- ¼ cup minced fresh basil
- 3 tablespoons grated Parmesan cheese
- 2 tablespoons lemon juice
- 1 tablespoon minced fresh parsley
- ¼ teaspoon white pepper
- ⅛ teaspoon ground nutmeg
- 8 cups packed fresh spinach, chopped
- Fresh lemon slices (optional)

1. Bring broth to a boil in medium saucepan over medium heat.
2. Beat egg substitute, basil, Parmesan cheese, lemon juice, parsley, white pepper and nutmeg in small bowl until well blended.
3. Stir spinach into broth; simmer 1 minute. Slowly pour egg mixture into broth mixture, whisking constantly so egg threads form. Simmer 2 to 3 minutes or until egg is cooked. Garnish with lemon slices. Serve immediately.

NOTE The soup may look curdled.

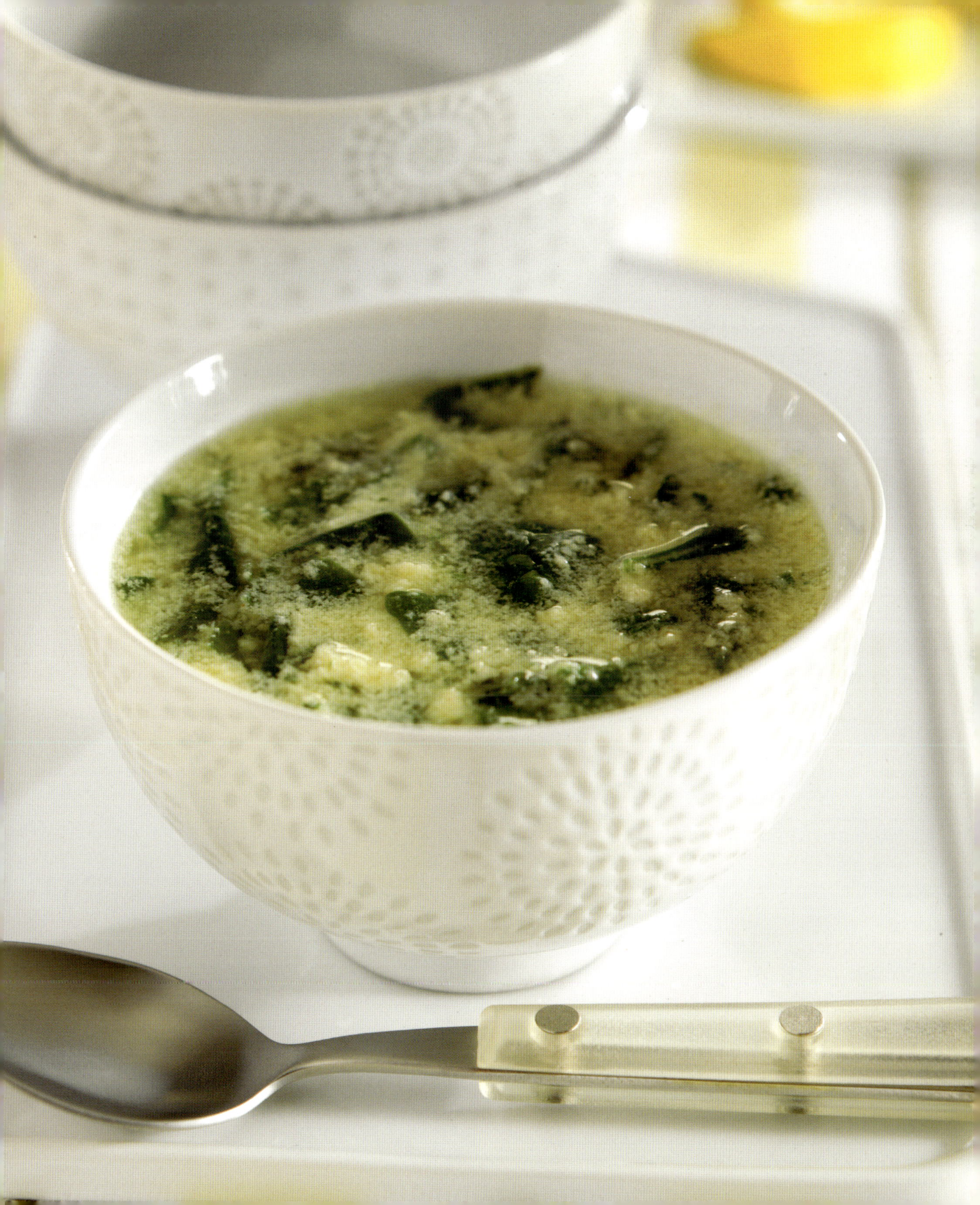

Spicy Sesame Noodles

makes 6 servings

- 6 ounces uncooked soba (buckwheat) noodles
- 2 teaspoons dark sesame oil
- 1 tablespoon sesame seeds
- ½ cup fat-free reduced-sodium chicken broth
- 1 tablespoon creamy peanut butter
- ¼ cup thinly sliced green onions
- ½ cup minced red bell pepper
- 4 teaspoons reduced-sodium soy sauce
- 1½ teaspoons finely chopped seeded jalapeño pepper*
- ¼ teaspoon red pepper flakes

***Jalapeño peppers can sting and irritate the skin, so wear rubber gloves when handling peppers and do not touch your eyes.**

1. Cook noodles according to package directions. (Do not overcook.) Rinse noodles thoroughly with cold running water; drain. Place noodles in large bowl; toss with oil.
2. Cook sesame seeds in small skillet over medium heat about 3 minutes or until seeds begin to pop and turn golden brown, stirring frequently. Remove from skillet.
3. Whisk broth and peanut butter in medium bowl until blended. (Mixture may look curdled.) Stir in green onions, bell pepper, soy sauce, jalapeño pepper and red pepper flakes.
4. Pour sauce over noodles; toss to coat. Cover and let stand 30 minutes at room temperature or refrigerate up to 24 hours. Sprinkle with toasted sesame seeds before serving.

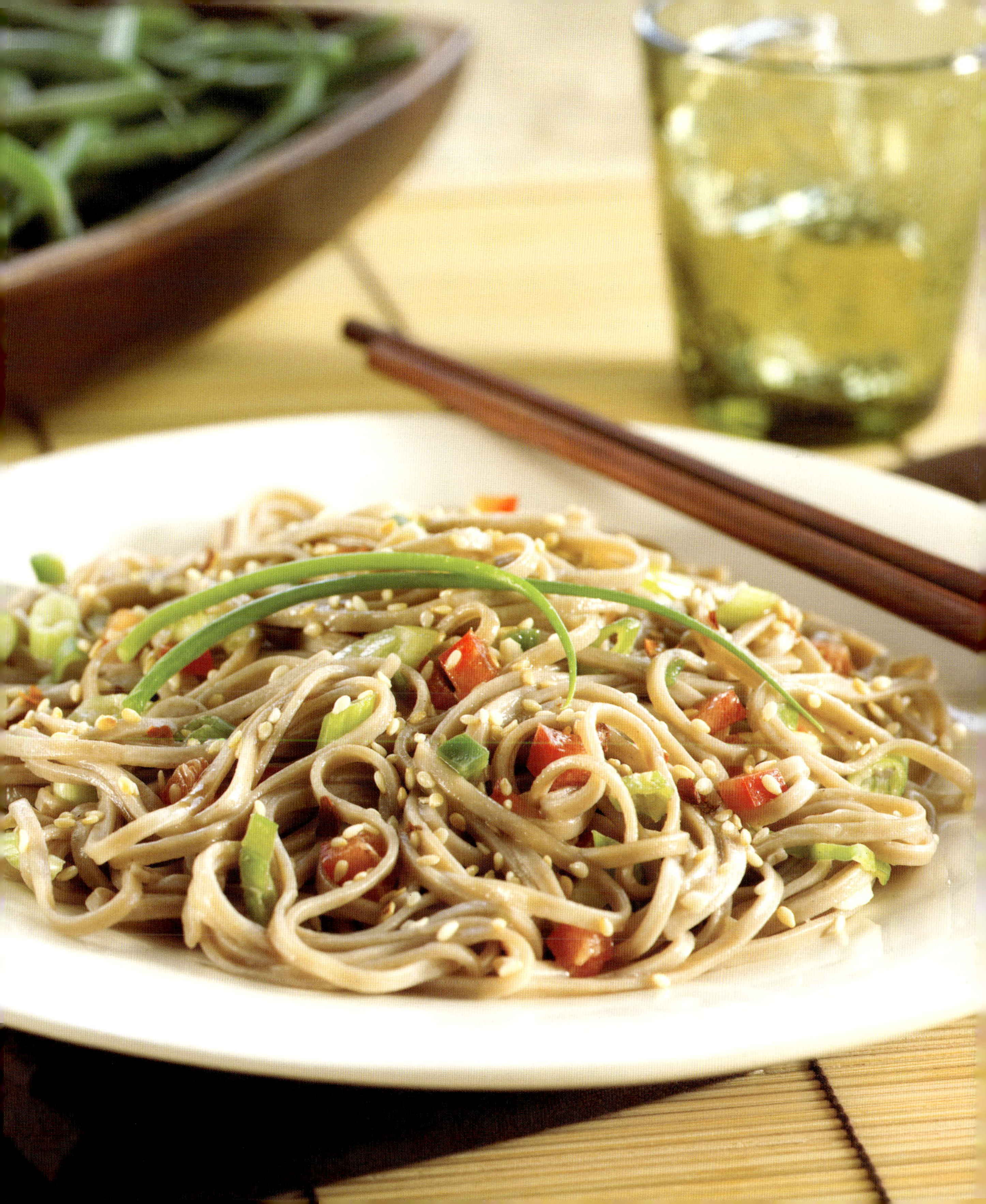

Italian Eggplant with Millet and Pepper Stuffing

makes 4 servings

- ¼ cup uncooked millet
- 2 small eggplants (about 12 ounces total)
- ¼ cup chopped red bell pepper, divided
- ¼ cup chopped green bell pepper, divided
- 1 teaspoon olive oil
- 1½ cups fat-free reduced-sodium vegetable broth
- ½ teaspoon ground cumin
- ½ teaspoon dried oregano
- ⅛ teaspoon red pepper flakes

1. Cook and stir millet in large heavy skillet over medium heat 5 minutes or until golden brown. Transfer to small bowl; set aside.
2. Slice eggplants in half lengthwise. Scoop out flesh, leaving ¼-inch shell. Finely chop seggplant. Combine 1 tablespoon red bell pepper and 1 tablespoon green bell pepper in small bowl; set aside.
3. Heat oil in same skillet over medium heat. Add chopped eggplant and remaining red and green bell pepper; cook and stir about 8 minutes or until eggplant is tender.
4. Stir in toasted millet, broth, cumin, oregano and red pepper flakes. Bring to a boil over high heat. Reduce heat to medium-low; cover and cook 35 minutes or until liquid is absorbed and millet is tender. Remove from heat; let stand, covered, 10 minutes.
5. Preheat oven to 350°F. Pour 1 cup water into 8-inch square baking pan. Fill eggplant shells with eggplant-millet mixture. Sprinkle with reserved chopped bell peppers, pressing in lightly. Carefully place filled eggplants in prepared pan. Bake 15 minutes or until heated through.

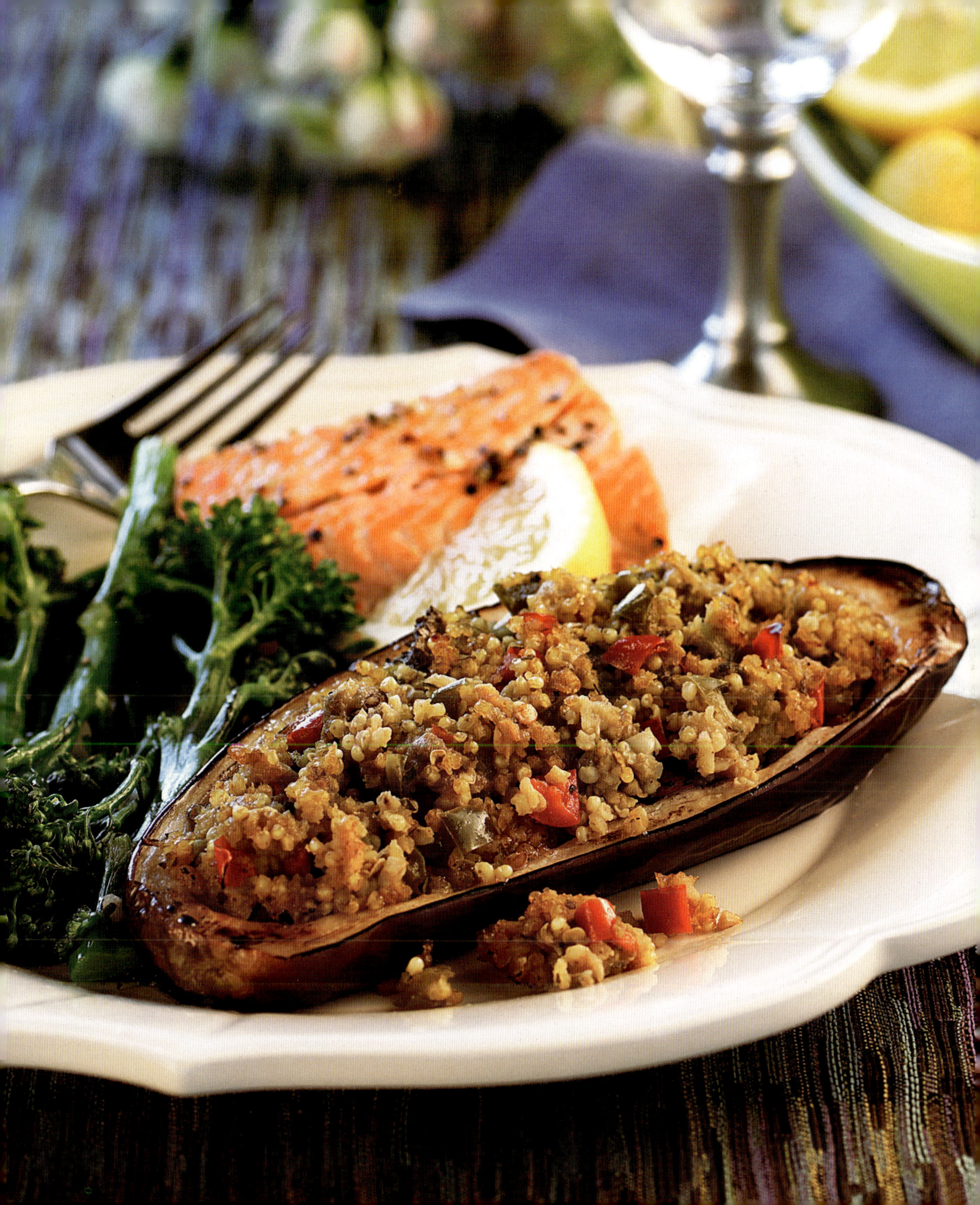

Quinoa and Vegetable Medley

makes 6 servings

- 2 medium sweet potatoes, cut into ½-inch-thick slices
- 1 medium eggplant, peeled and cut into ½-inch cubes
- 1 medium tomato, cut into wedges
- 1 large green bell pepper, sliced
- 1 small onion, cut into wedges
- ½ teaspoon salt
- ¼ teaspoon black pepper
- ¼ teaspoon ground red pepper
- 1 cup uncooked quinoa
- ½ teaspoon dried thyme
- ¼ teaspoon dried marjoram
- 2 cups water or fat-free reduced-sodium vegetable broth

Slow Cooker Directions

1. Spray slow cooker with nonstick cooking spray. Combine sweet potatoes, eggplant, tomato, bell pepper, onion, salt, black pepper and ground red pepper in slow cooker; toss to coat.
2. Place quinoa in fine-mesh strainer; rinse well under cold running water. Add to vegetable mixture with thyme and marjoram. Stir in broth.
3. Cover; cook on LOW 5 hours or on HIGH 2½ hours until quinoa is tender and broth is absorbed.

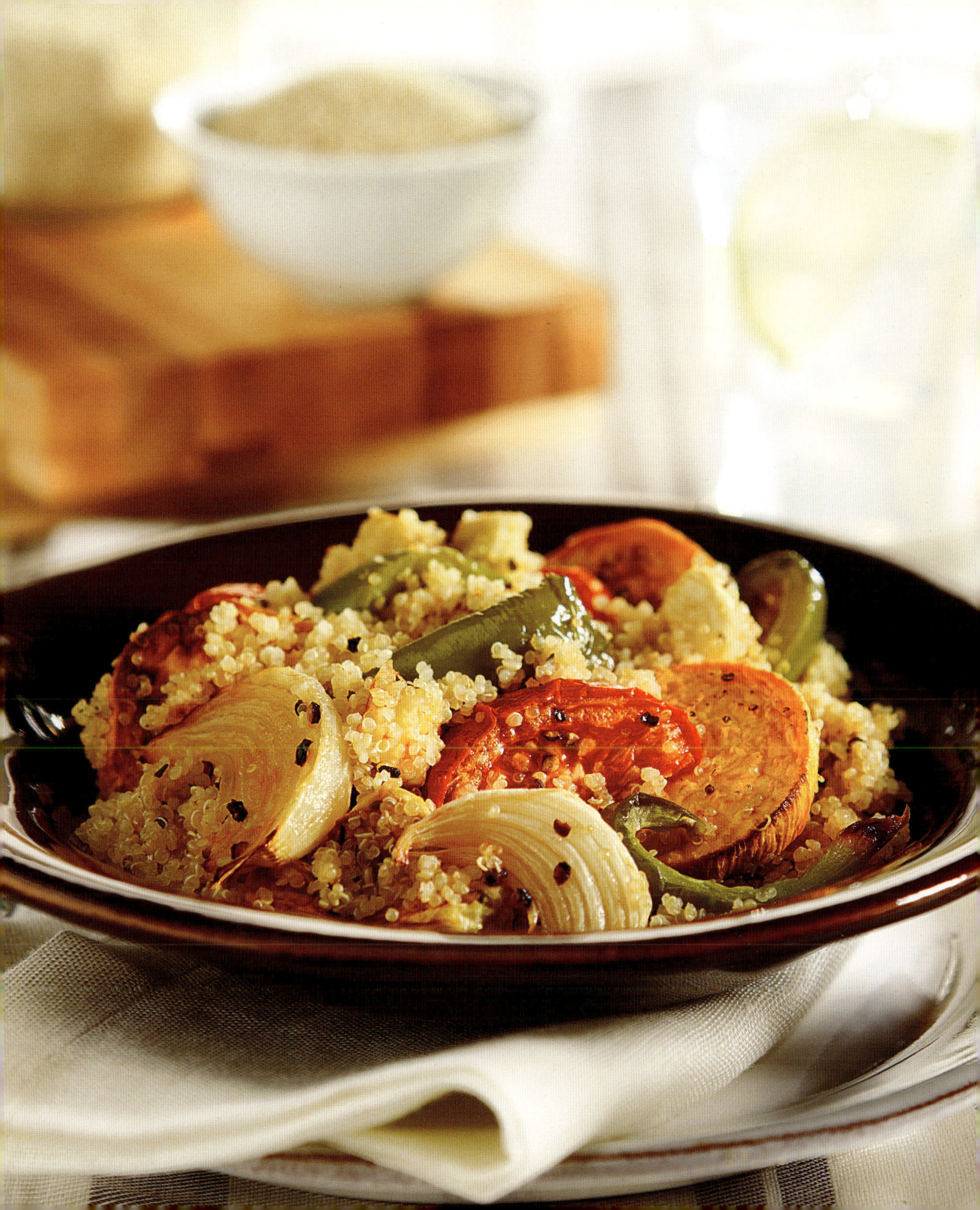

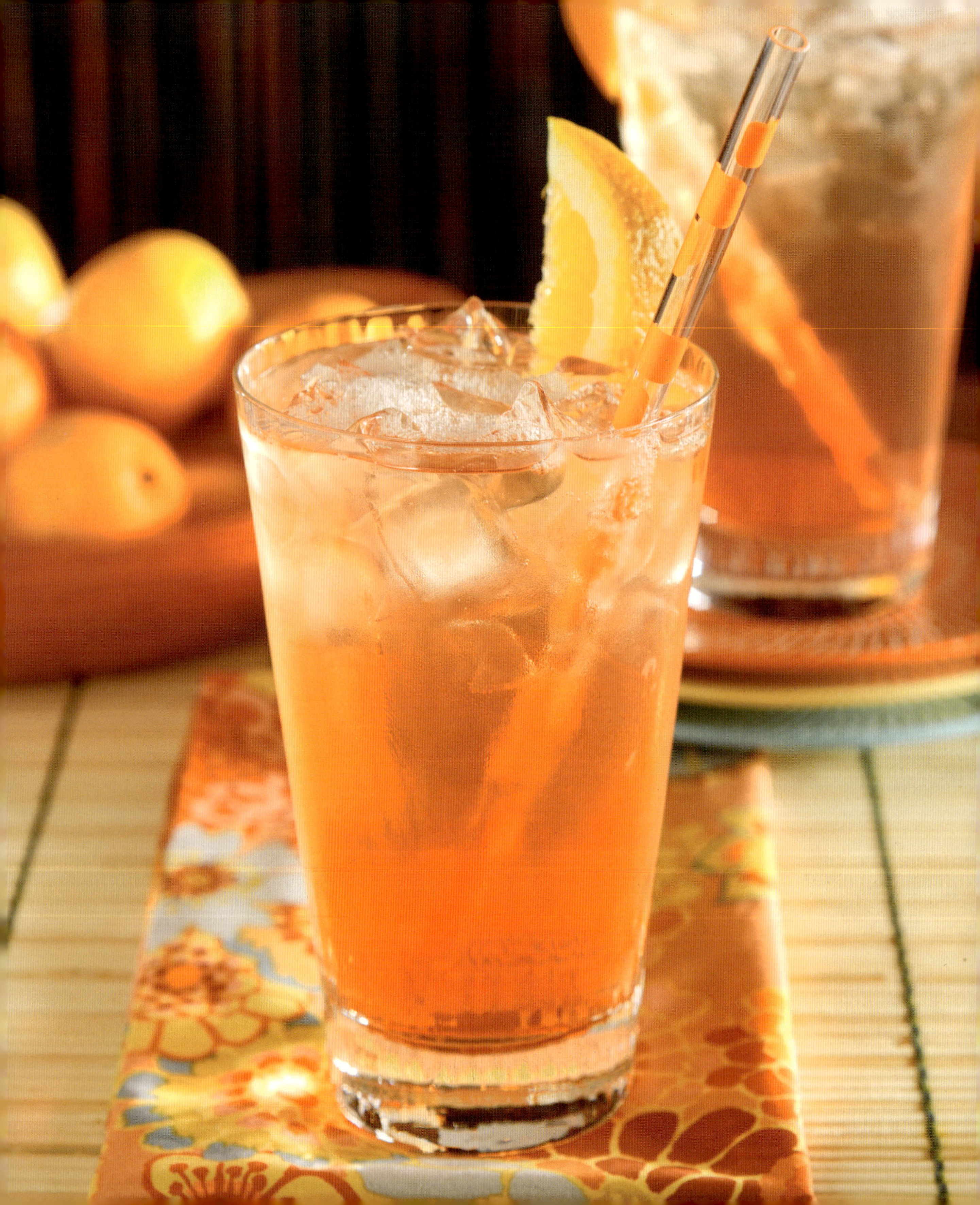

BEVERAGES & SMOOTHIES

Orange Tea Zinger

makes 2 servings

- 2 orange or tangerine-flavored herbal tea bags
- 1 cup boiling water
- Ice
- 2 cans (12 ounces each) unsweetened seltzer water

1. Steep both tea bags in boiling water about 4 minutes to brew 1 cup of double-strength tea. Remove tea bags and refrigerate until cool.
2. To serve, pour half of cooled tea (just less than ½ cup) over ice in each of two tall glasses. Fill glasses with seltzer water; stir gently to blend.

Go Green Smoothie

makes 1 serving

- 1½ cups ice cubes
- 1 cup packed torn spinach
- ½ cup vanilla almond milk
- ¼ cup vanilla low-fat yogurt
- ¼ avocado
- 1 teaspoon lemon juice

Combine ice, spinach, milk, yogurt, avocado and lemon juice in blender; blend until smooth.

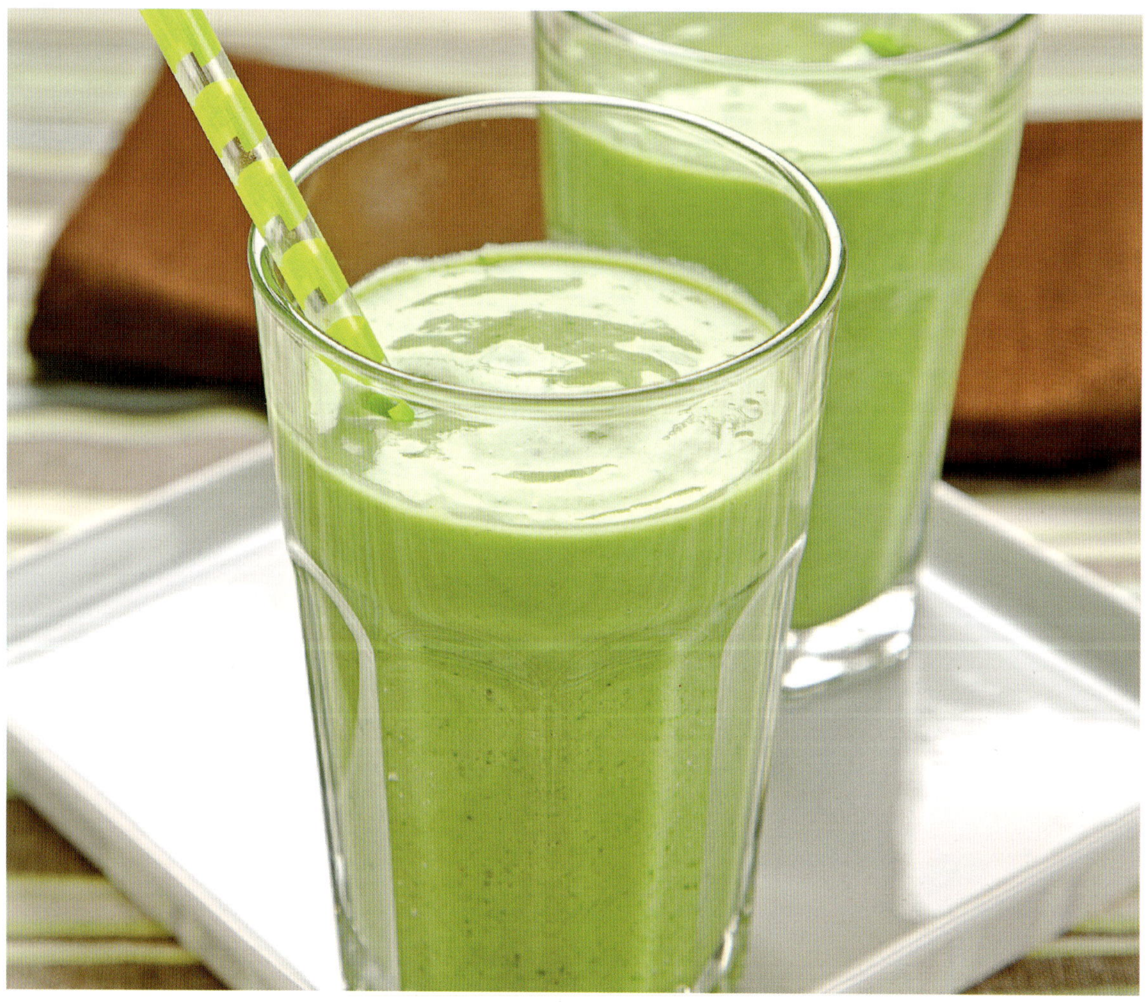

Refresh Smoothie

makes 2 servings

- ½ cucumber, peeled and seeded
- 1 cup frozen mixed berries
- Ice cubes
- 4 teaspoons sugar
- Grated peel and juice of 1 lime

Combine cucumber, berries, ice, sugar, lime peel and lime juice in blender; blend until smooth.

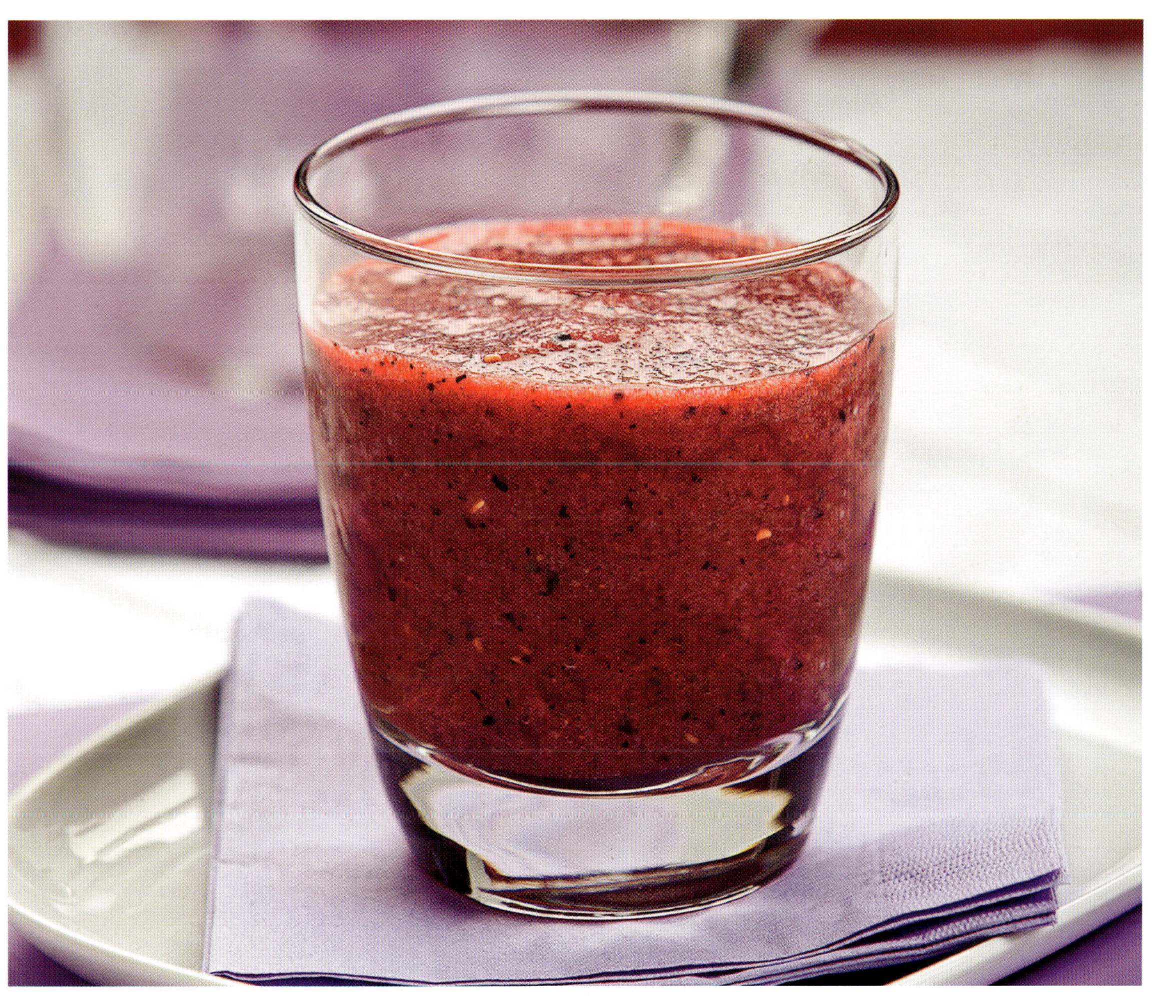

Cool Cucumber

makes 2 servings

- **1 cucumber**
- **¼ pineapple, peeled**
- **¼ cup fresh cilantro**

Juice cucumber, pineapple and cilantro. Stir.

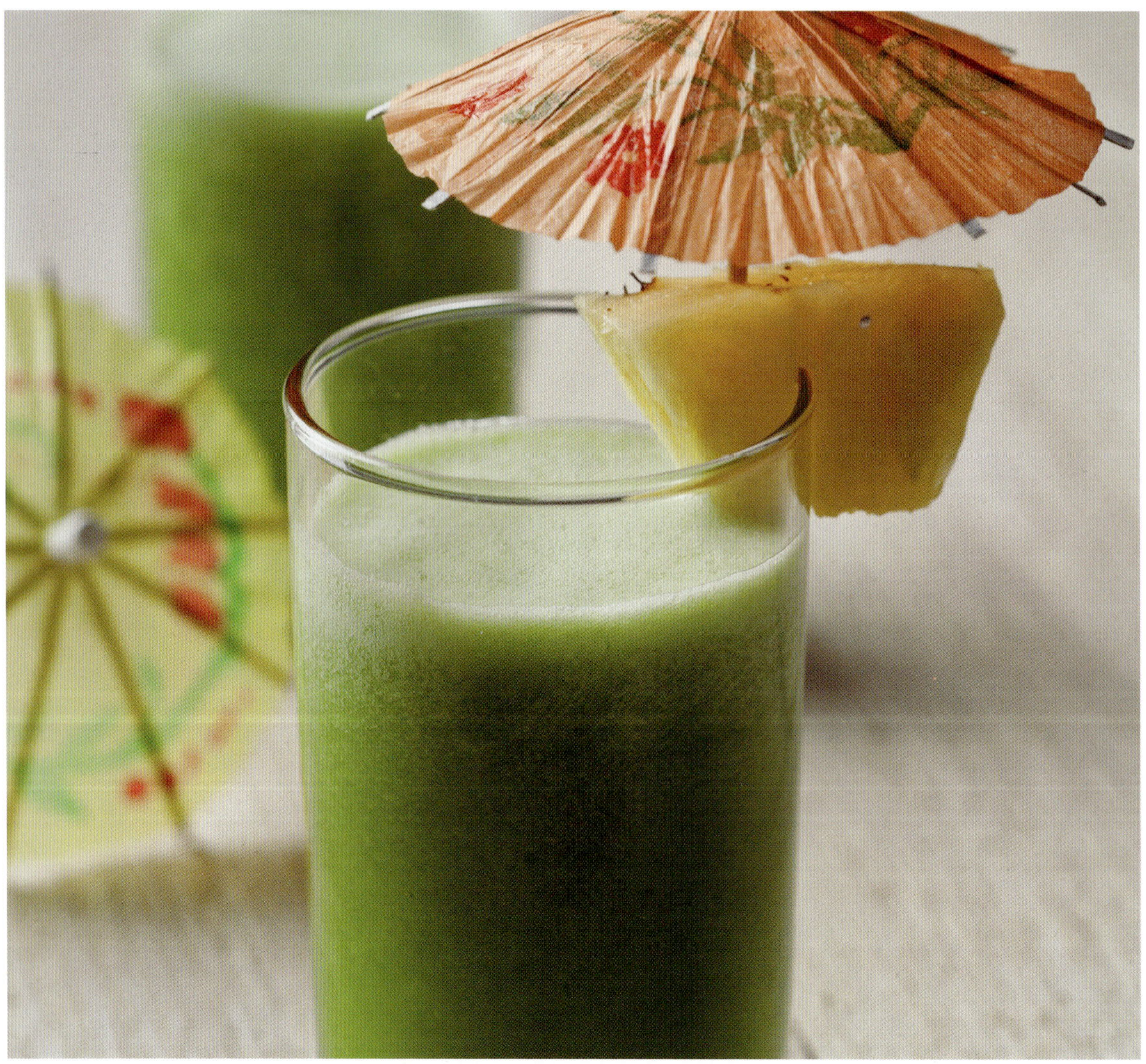

Bedtime Cocktail

makes 2 servings

- ½ head romaine lettuce
- 2 stalks celery
- ½ cucumber

Juice romaine, celery and cucumber. Stir.

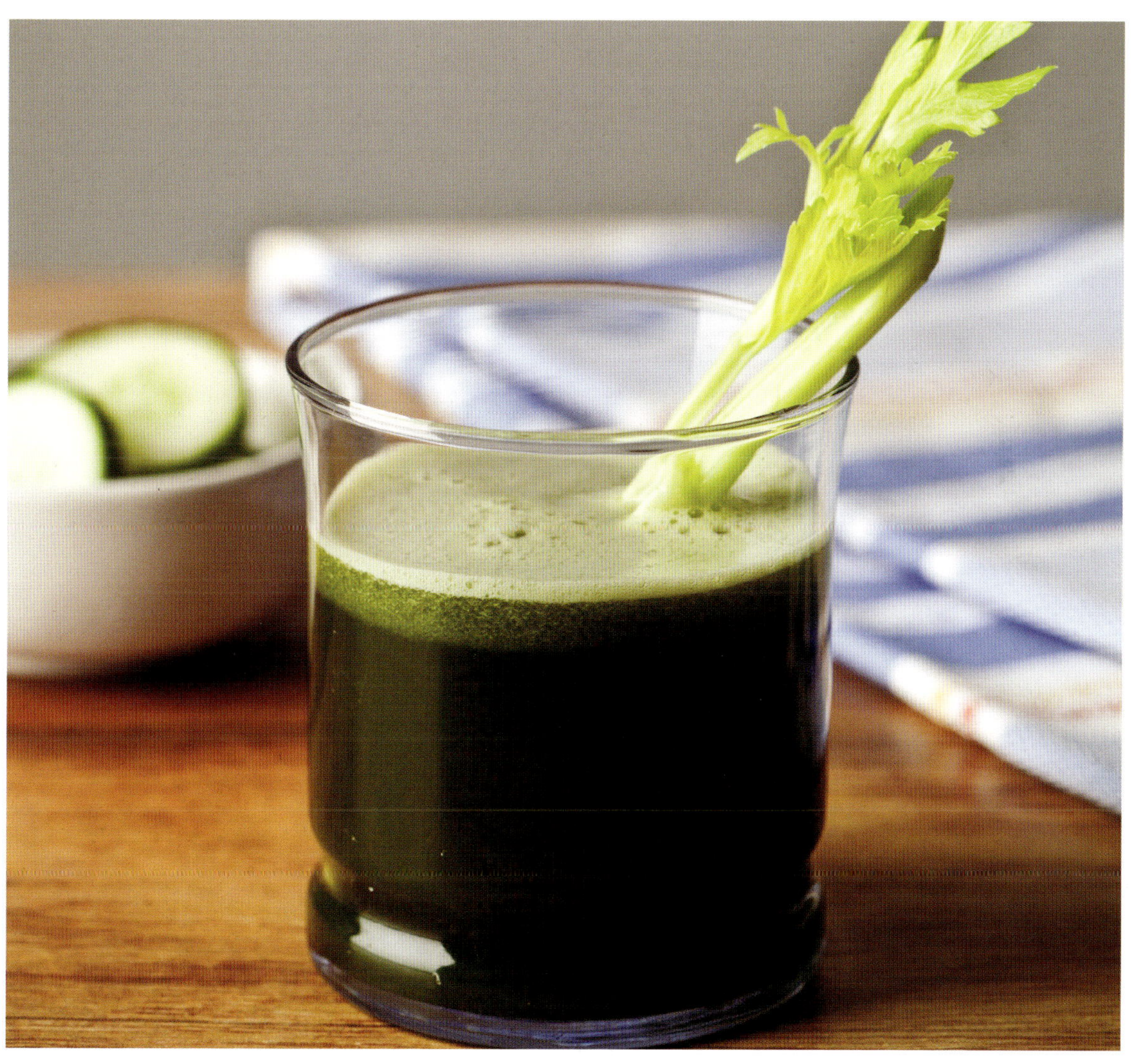

Fiery Cucumber Beet Juice

makes 2 servings

1 cucumber

1 beet

1 lemon, peeled

1 inch fresh ginger, peeled

½ jalapeño pepper*

Jalapeño peppers can sting and irritate the skin, so wear rubber gloves when handling peppers and do not touch your eyes.

Juice cucumber, beet, lemon, ginger and jalapeño pepper. Stir.

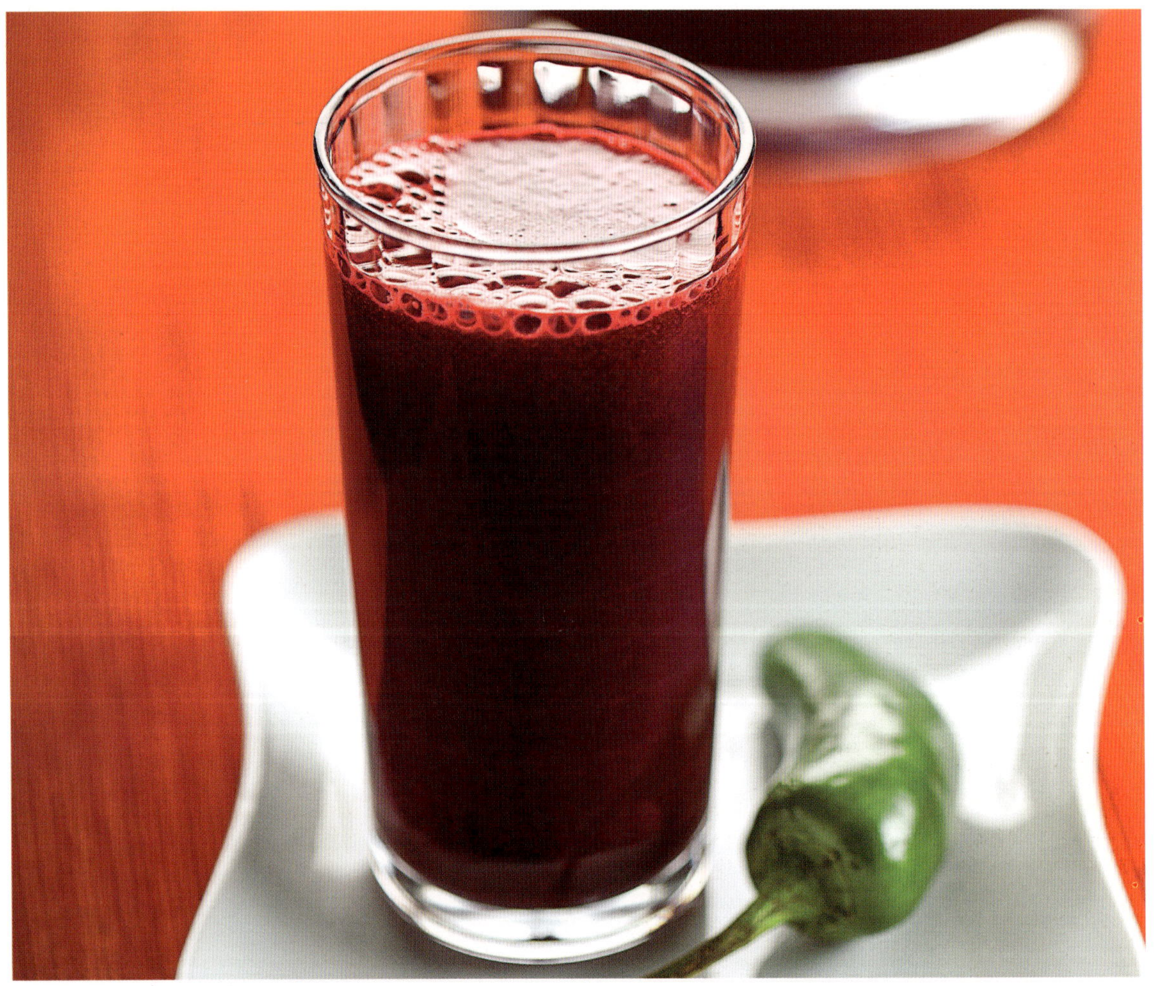

Spiced Pumpkin Banana Smoothie

makes 1 serving

- ½ cup almond milk
- ½ frozen banana
- ½ cup unsweetened canned pumpkin
- ½ cup ice cubes
- 1 teaspoon ground flaxseeds
- ¼ teaspoon ground cinnamon
- ⅛ teaspoon ground ginger
- Dash ground nutmeg

Combine almond milk, banana, pumpkin, ice, flaxseeds, cinnamon, ginger and nutmeg in blender; blend until smooth.

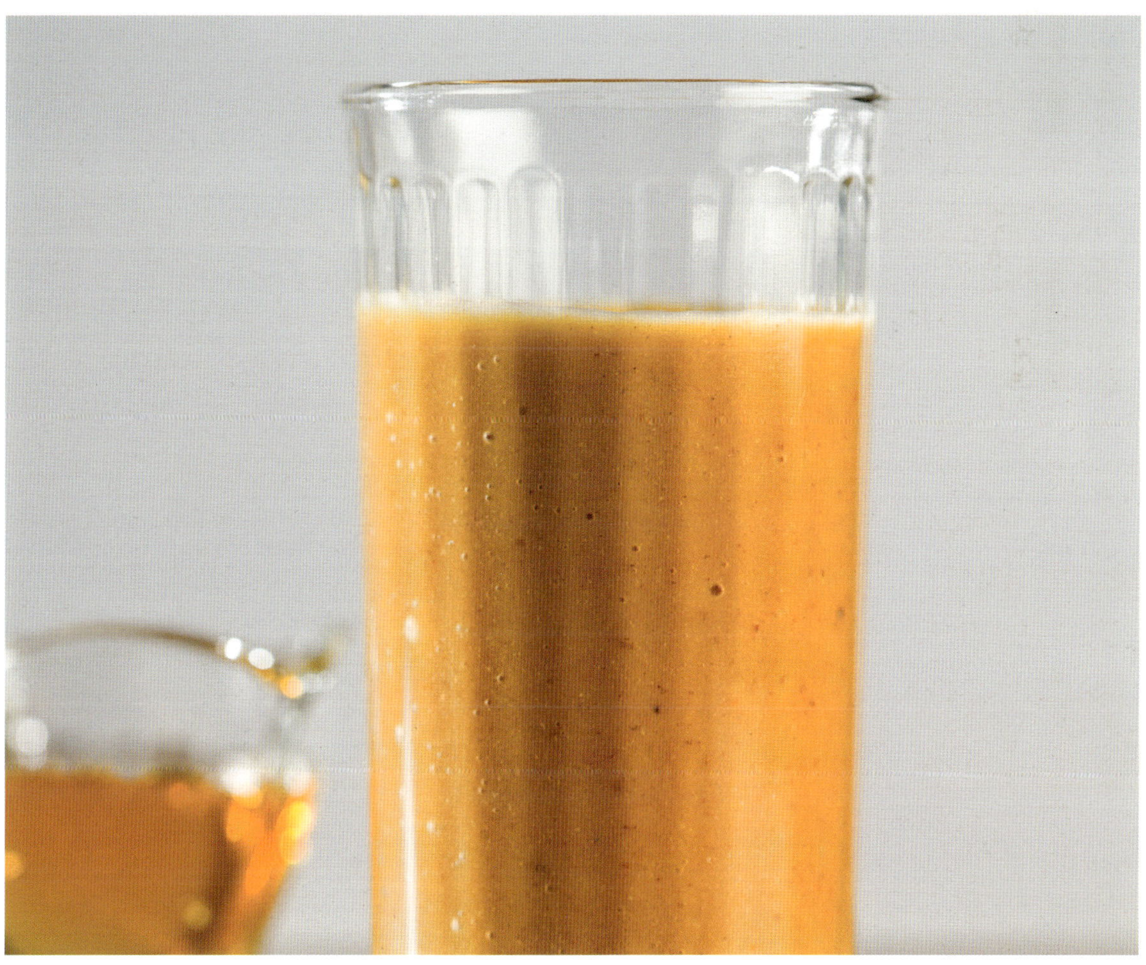

Cleansing Green Juice

makes 2 servings

- **4 leaves bok choy**
- **1 stalk celery**
- **½ cucumber**
- **¼ bulb fennel**
- **½ lemon, peeled**

Juice bok choy, celery, cucumber, fennel and lemon. Stir.

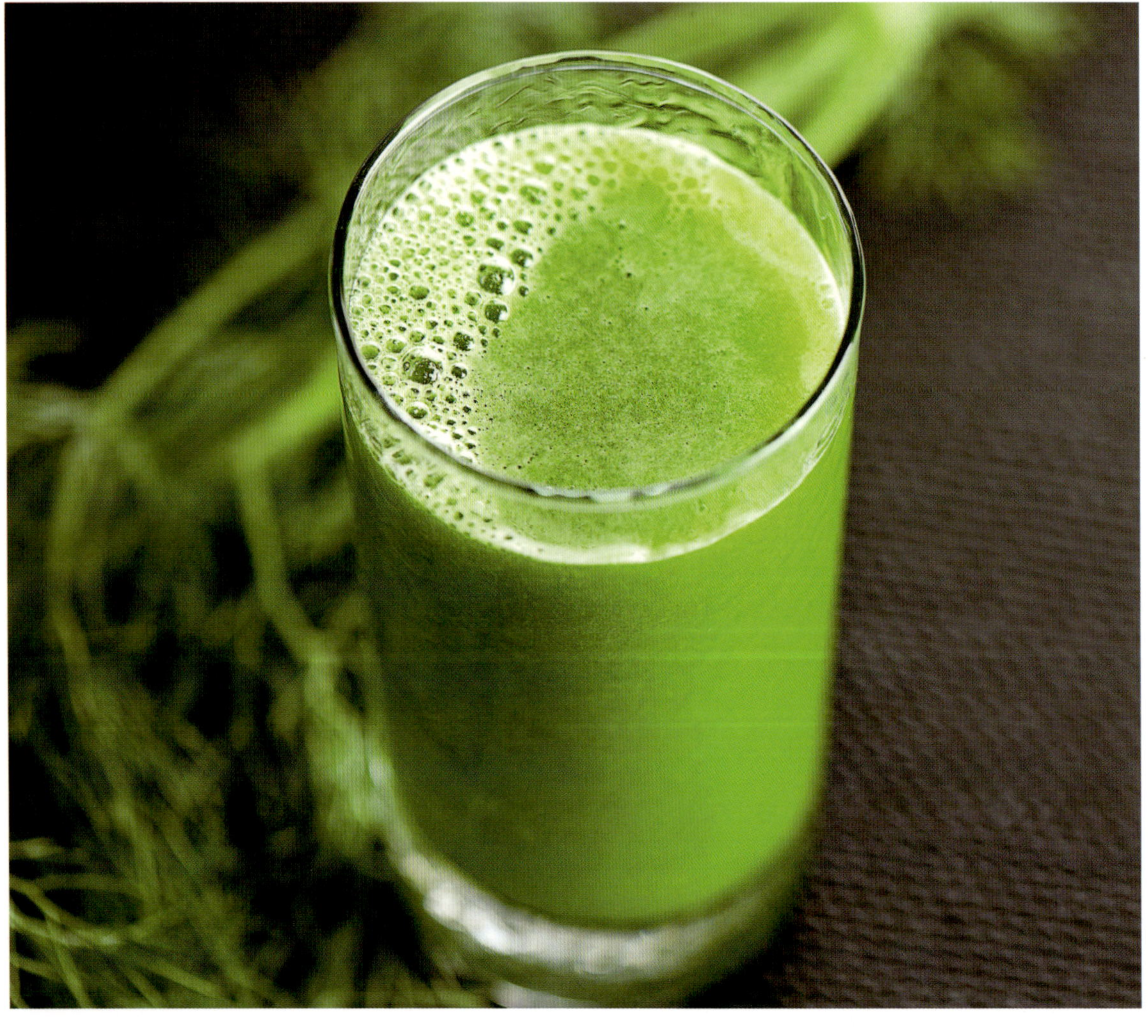

Double Green Pineapple

makes 1 serving

- 4 leaves Swiss chard
- 4 leaves kale
- ¼ pineapple, peeled

Juice chard, kale and pineapple. Stir.

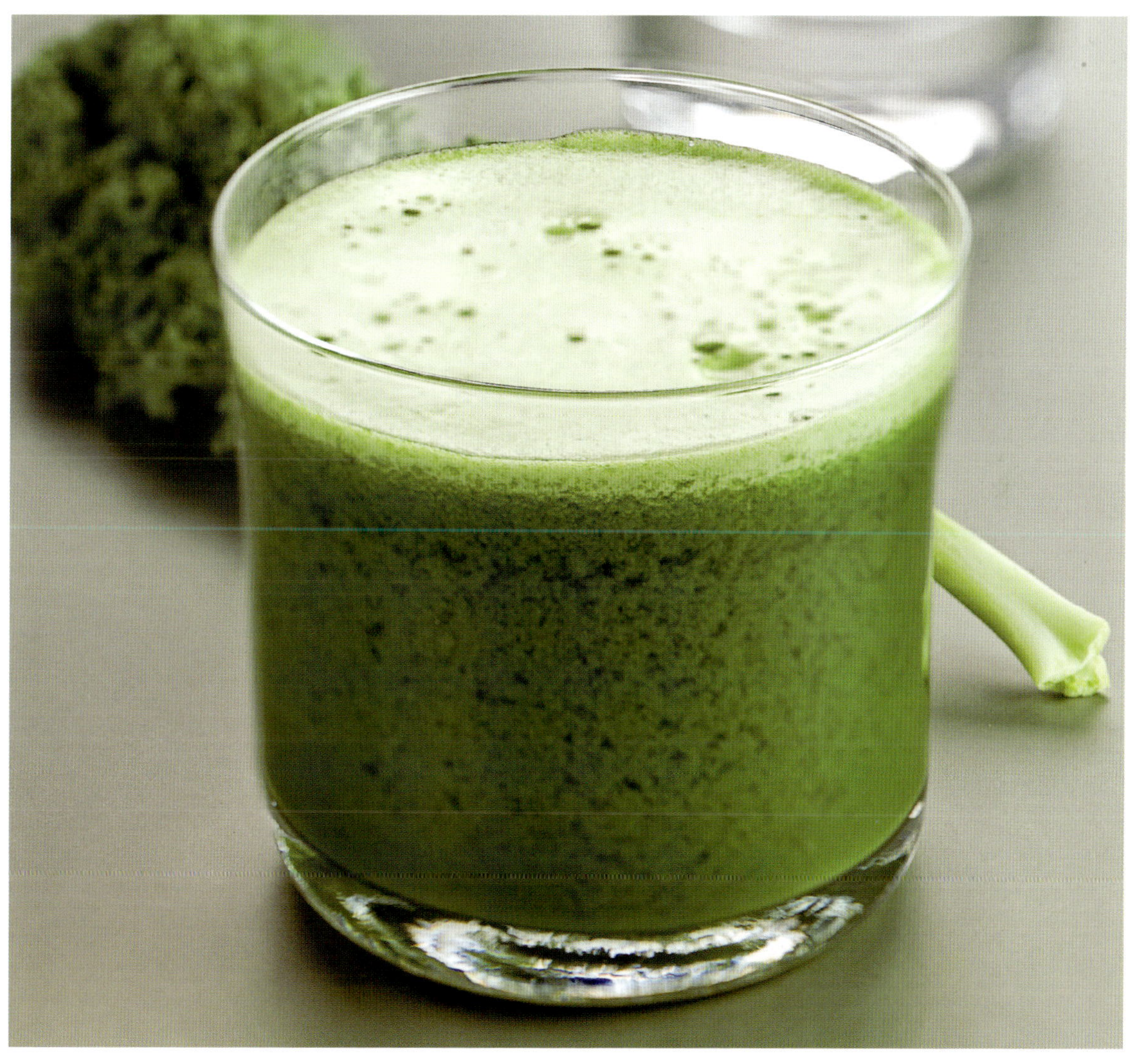

Ginger-Lime Iced Green Tea

makes 4 servings

1 quart water
2 thin slices fresh ginger (about 1 inch in diameter)
4 green tea bags
¼ cup lime juice (2 to 3 limes)
Ice cubes
Lime slices (optional)

1. Bring water and ginger to a boil in large saucepan. Pour water over tea bags in teapot or 4-cup heatproof measuring cup; steep 3 minutes. Remove and discard tea bags and ginger. Cool tea to room temperature.
2. Add lime juice to tea; pour into four ice-filled glasses. Sweeten with sugar substitute, such as stevia, if desired. Garnish with lime slices.

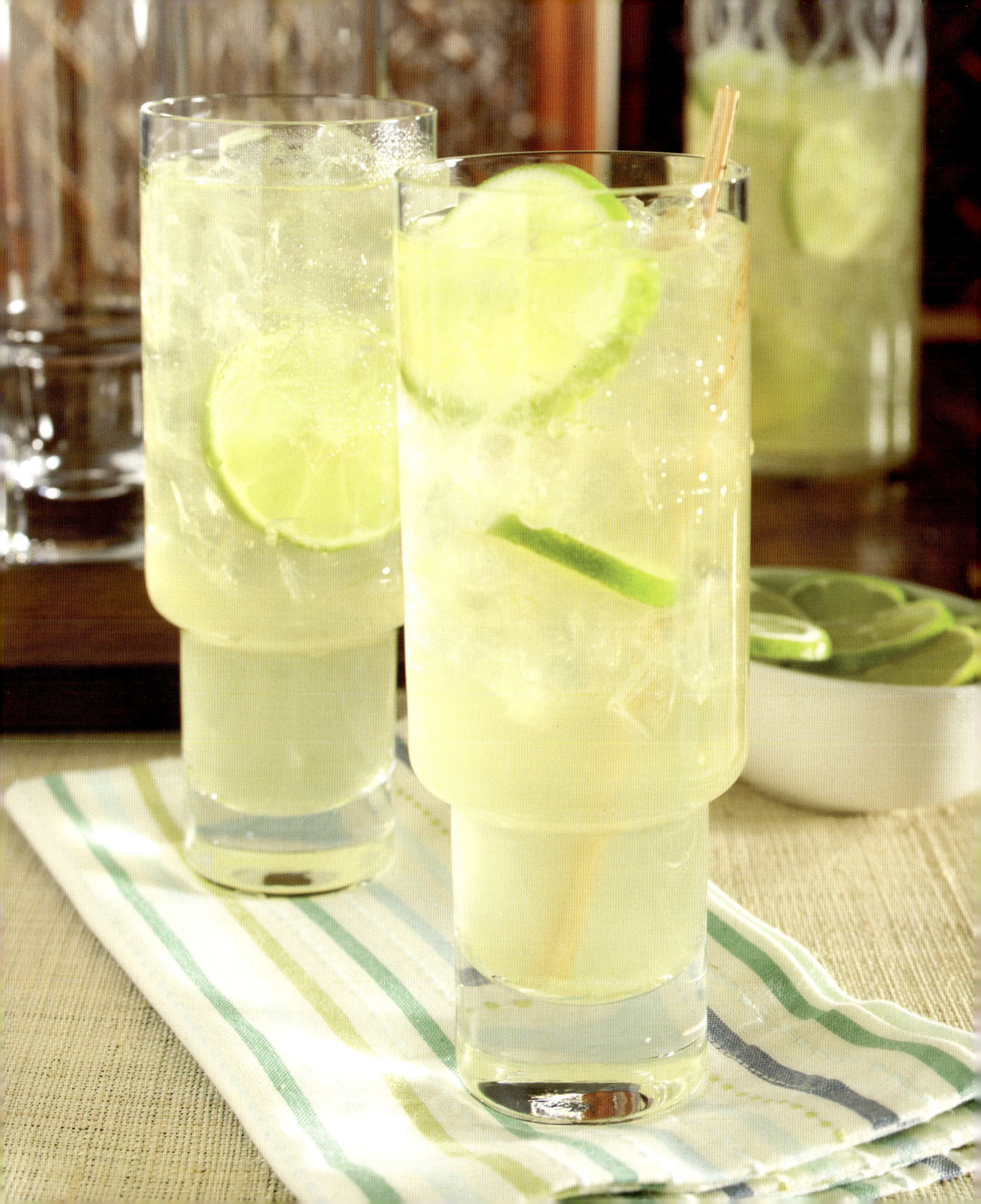

Cucumber Punch

makes 10 to 12 servings

- **1 English cucumber, thinly sliced**
- **1 cup water**
- **4 ounces thawed frozen limeade concentrate**
- **1 bottle (1 liter) club soda, chilled**
- **Ice cubes**
- **Lime wedges (optional)**

1. Combine cucumber slices, water and limeade concentrate in punch bowl or pitcher. Refrigerate 1 hour.
2. Add club soda and ice just before serving. Garnish with lime wedges.

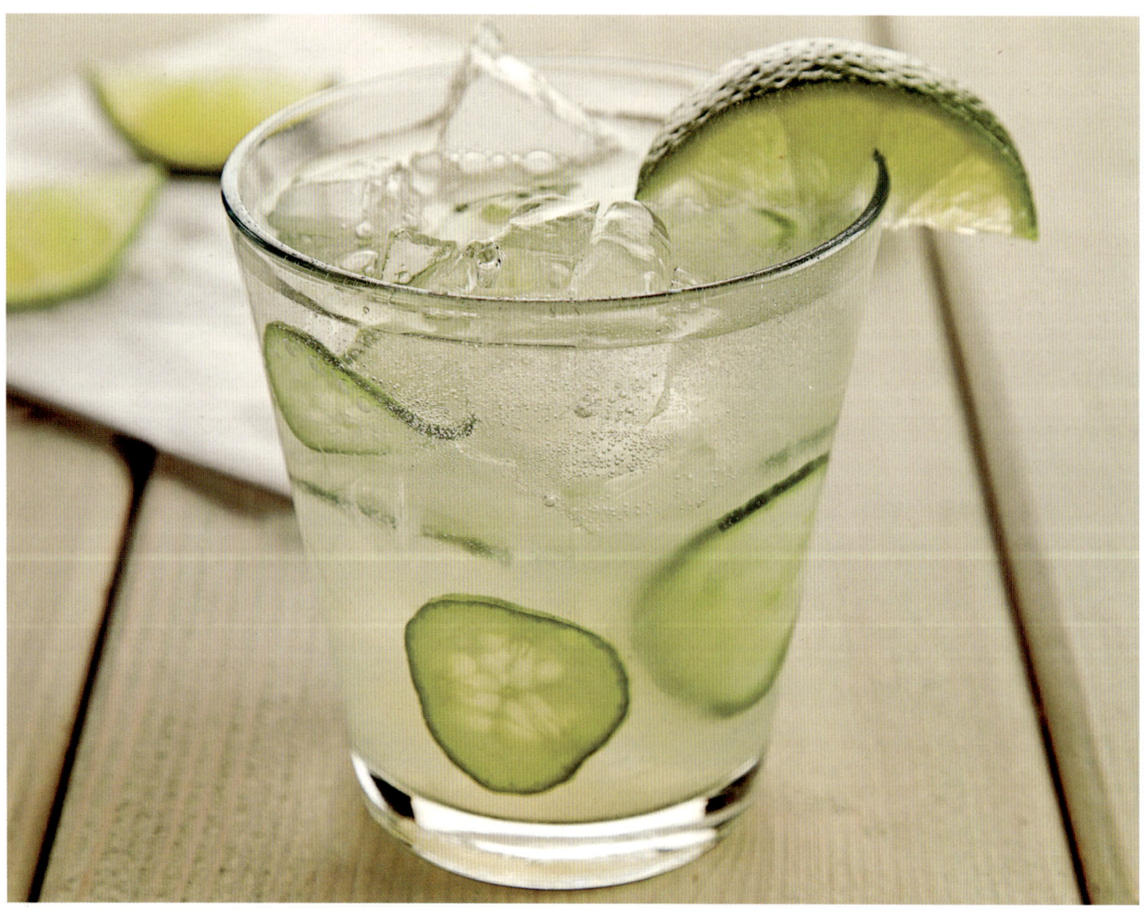

Simple Raspberry Smoothie

makes 2 servings

- **½ cup unsweetened coconut milk**
- **1 cup fresh raspberries**
- **½ cup ice cubes**

Combine coconut milk, raspberries and ice in blender; blend until smooth.

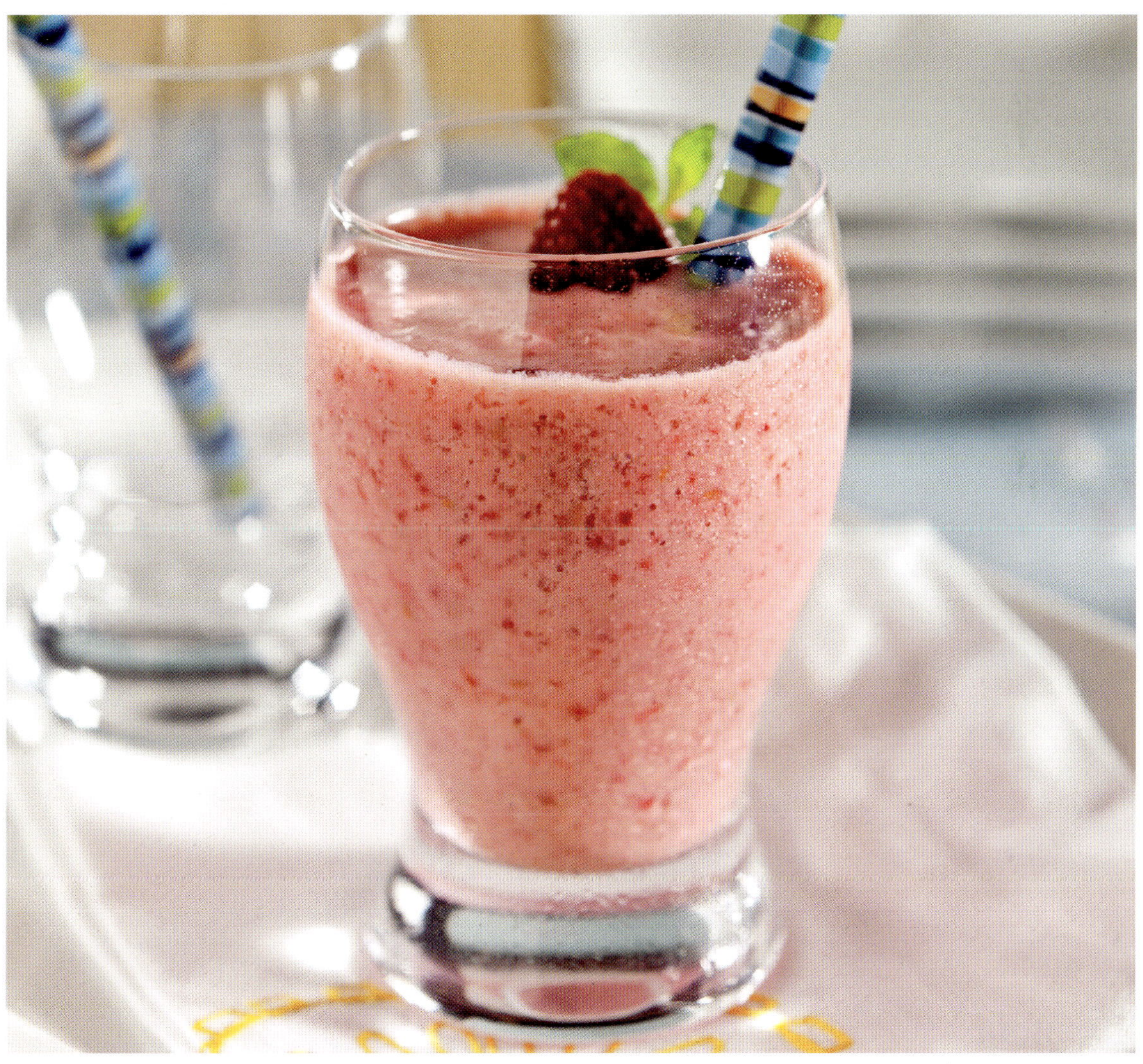

Chocolate Blueberry Shake

makes 1 serving

- ¼ cup unsweetened almond milk
- ½ cup fresh blueberries
- ¼ cup ice cubes
- ½ teaspoon unsweetened cocoa powder

Combine milk, blueberries, ice and cocoa in blender; blend until smooth.

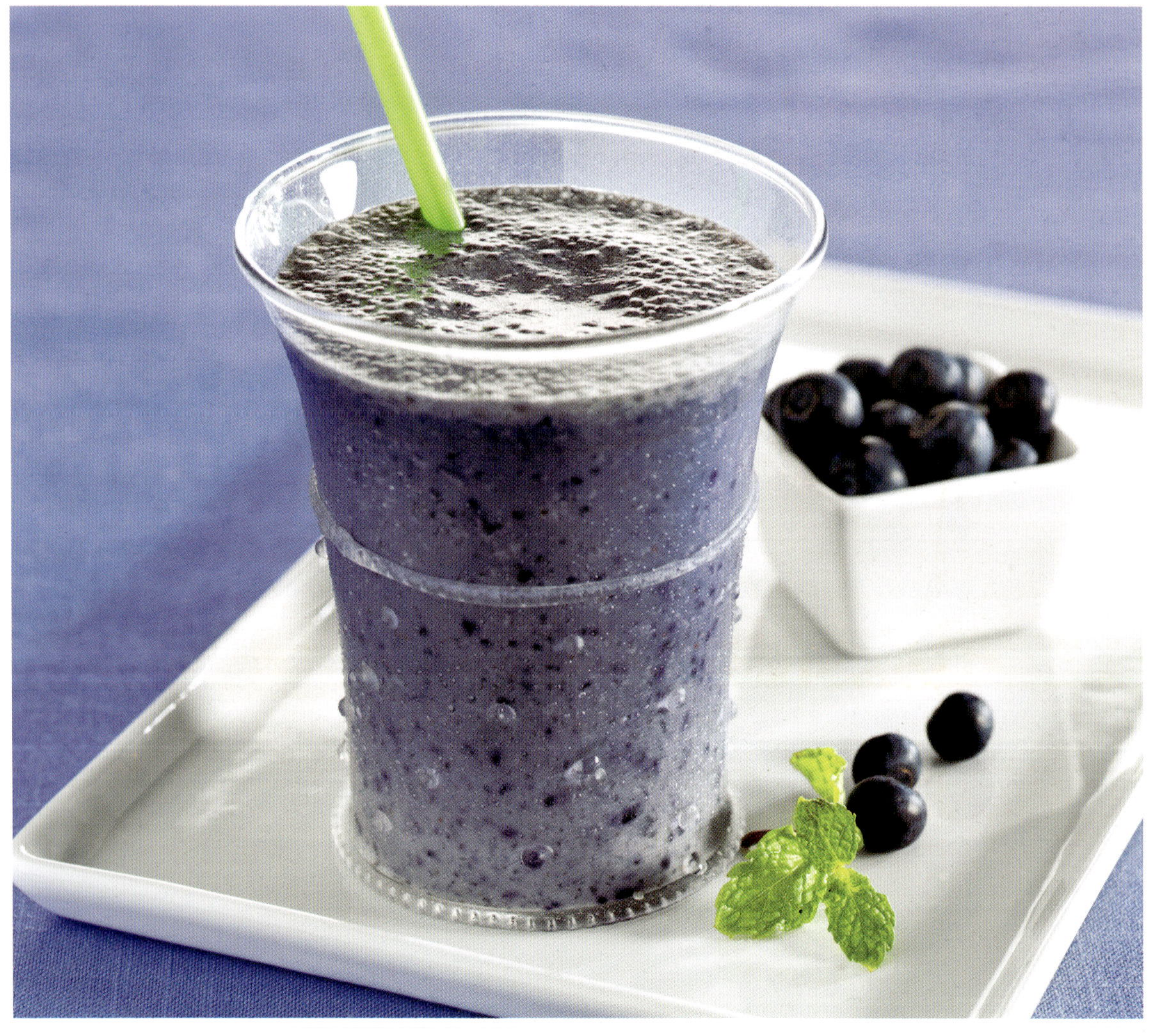

Blue Kale Smoothie

makes 2 servings

- ¼ **cup unsweetened almond milk**
- 1 **frozen banana**
- 1 **cup chopped fresh kale**
- ¼ **cup fresh blueberries**
- ¼ **cup ice cubes**

Combine milk, banana, kale, blueberries and ice in blender; blend until smooth.

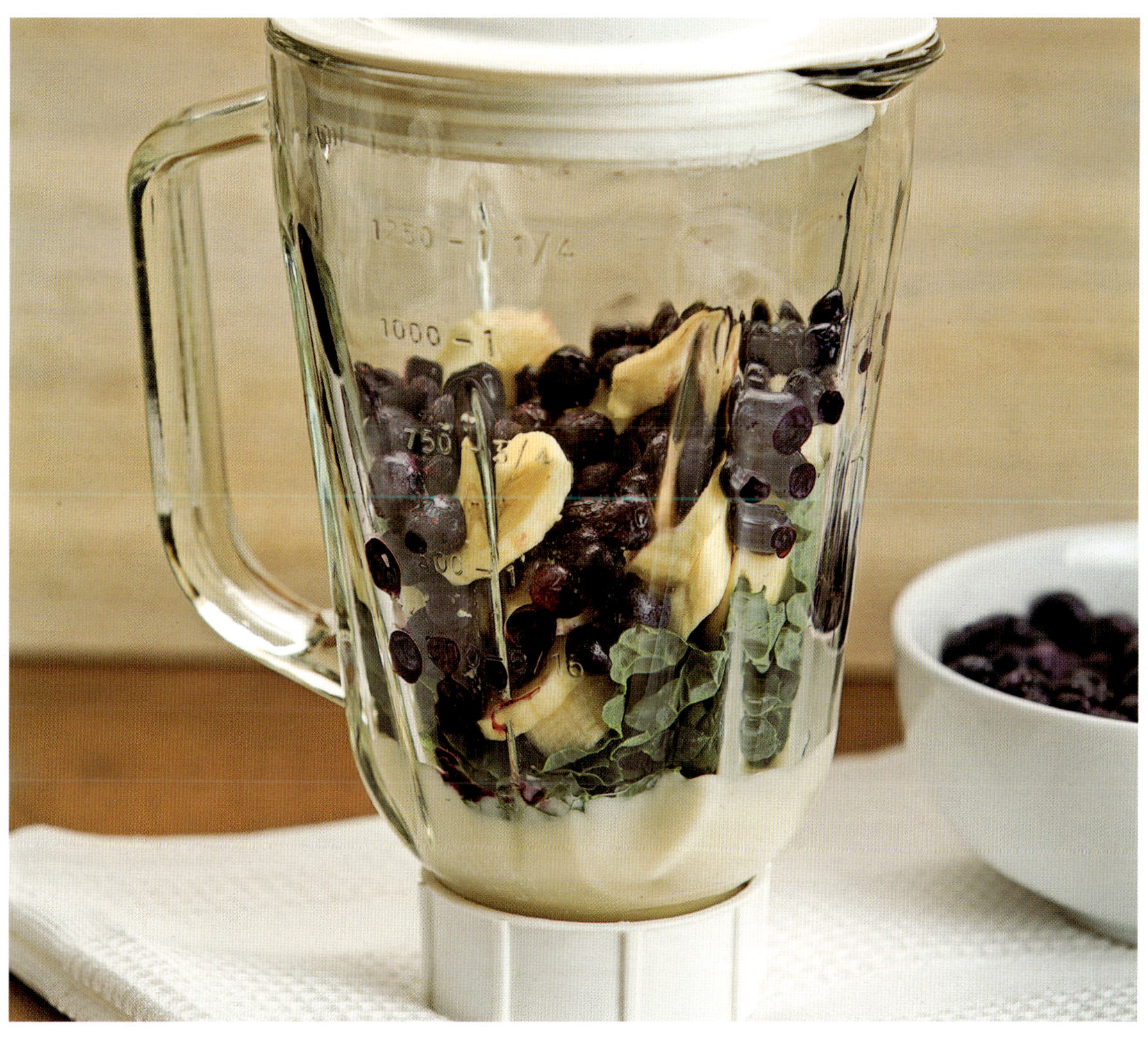

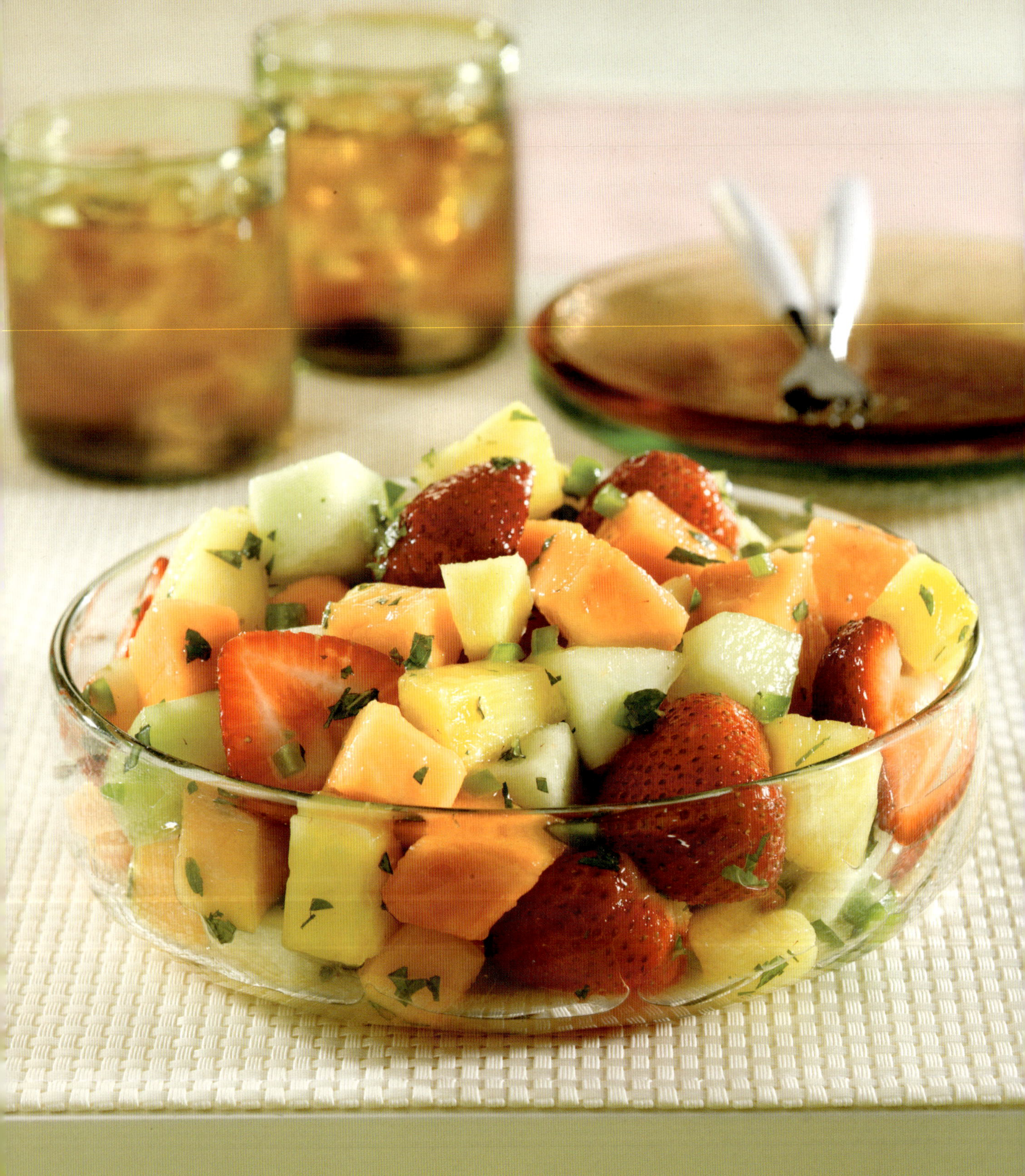

SNACKS & SWEETS

Hot and Spicy Fruit Salad

makes 8 servings

- ⅓ cup orange juice
- 3 tablespoons lime juice
- 3 tablespoons minced fresh mint, basil or cilantro, plus additional for garnish
- 2 jalapeño peppers,* seeded and minced
- ½ small honeydew melon, cut into cubes
- 1 pint fresh strawberries, stemmed, halved
- 1 cup fresh pineapple cubes

***Jalapeño peppers can sting and irritate the skin, so wear rubber gloves when handling peppers and do not touch your eyes.**

1. Blend orange juice, lime juice, 3 tablespoons mint and jalapeño peppers in small bowl.
2. Combine melon, strawberries and pineapple in large bowl. Pour orange juice mixture over fruit; toss gently until well blended.
3. Serve immediately or cover and refrigerate up to 3 hours. Garnish with fresh mint, if desired.

Toasted Coconut Quinoa Balls

makes 24 servings

½ cup uncooked quinoa
1 cup water
2 cups sweetened flaked coconut (about ½ of 14-ounce package), divided
½ cup creamy almond butter
1 tablespoon maple syrup
½ teaspoon ground cinnamon
½ teaspoon vanilla

1. Preheat oven to 350°F. Place quinoa in fine-mesh strainer; rinse well under cold running water.
2. Bring 1 cup water and quinoa in medium saucepan to a boil over high heat. Reduce heat to low; cover and simmer 10 to 15 minutes or until quinoa is tender and water is absorbed. Cool slightly.
3. Meanwhile, spread coconut in shallow baking pan. Bake 7 to 10 minutes or until lightly brown and toasted, stirring frequently. Cool slightly.
4. Combine quinoa, 1¼ cups coconut, almond butter, maple syrup, cinnamon and vanilla in medium bowl.
5. Shape mixture into 1-inch balls. Roll in remaining ¾ cup coconut to coat. Store leftovers in refrigerator.

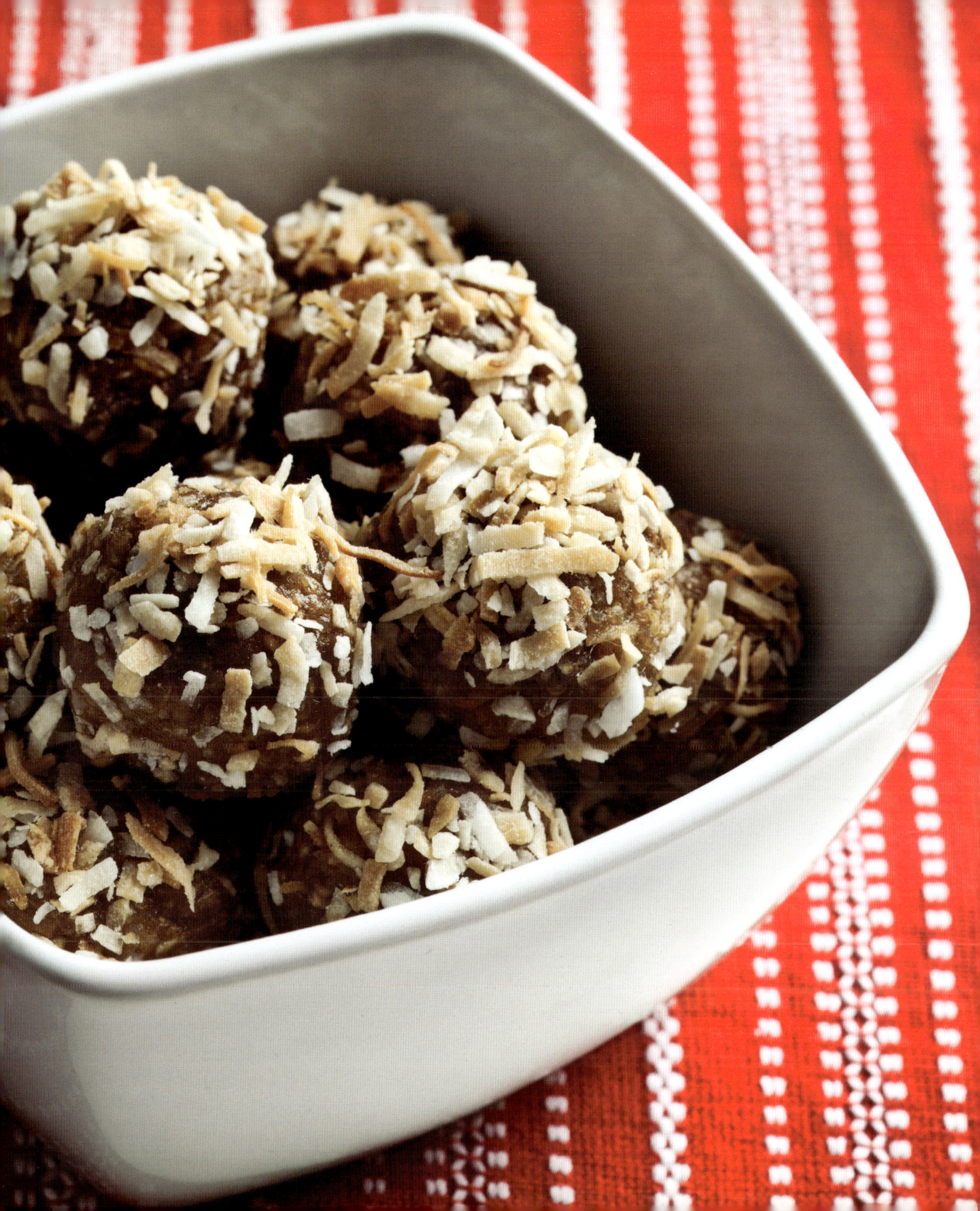

Kiwi and Strawberries with Pine Nuts

makes 4 servings

- **2 kiwi fruits**
- **1½ cups fresh strawberries**
- **1 tablespoon orange juice**
- **1 tablespoon pine nuts or pistachio nuts, toasted (see Tip)**

1. Peel kiwis and slice into thin rounds. Arrange on four dessert plates.
2. Wash, hull and slice strawberries. Arrange over kiwi slices. Drizzle orange juice evenly over each dish. Sprinkle with pine nuts.

TIP To toast pine nuts, cook them in a small skillet over medium heat 1 to 2 minutes or until lightly browned, stirring frequently.

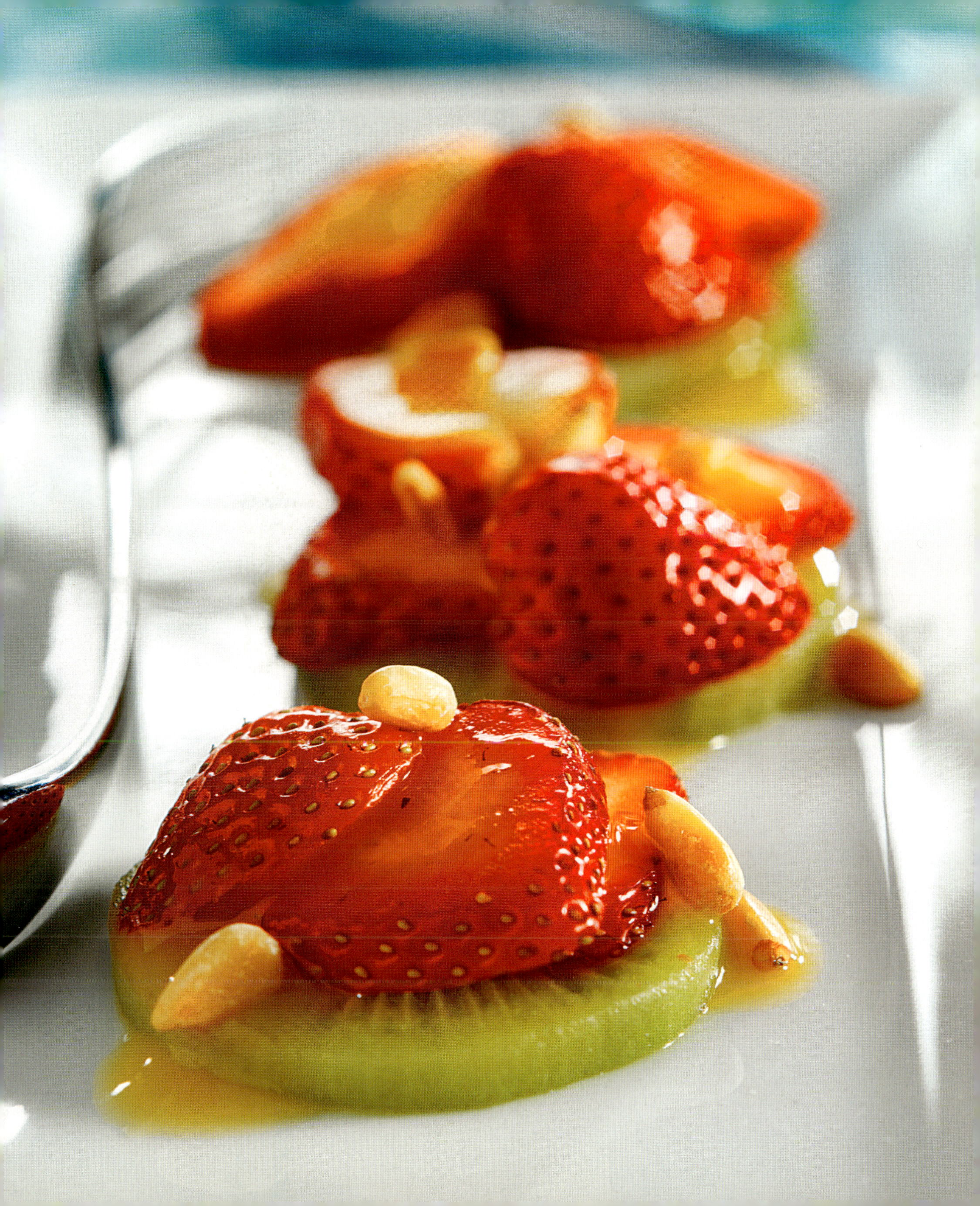

Spicy Roasted Chickpeas

makes 4 servings

- 1 can (about 15 ounces) chickpeas, rinsed and drained
- 3 tablespoons olive oil
- ½ teaspoon salt
- ½ teaspoon black pepper
- ¾ to 1 tablespoon chili powder
- ⅛ to ¼ teaspoon ground red pepper
- 1 lime, cut into wedges

1. Preheat oven to 400°F.
2. Combine chickpeas, oil, salt and black pepper in large bowl; toss to coat. Spread in single layer on 15×10-inch jelly-roll pan.
3. Bake 15 minutes or until chickpeas begin to brown, shaking pan twice.
4. Sprinkle with chili powder and ground red pepper. Roast 5 minutes or until dark golden brown. Serve with lime wedges.

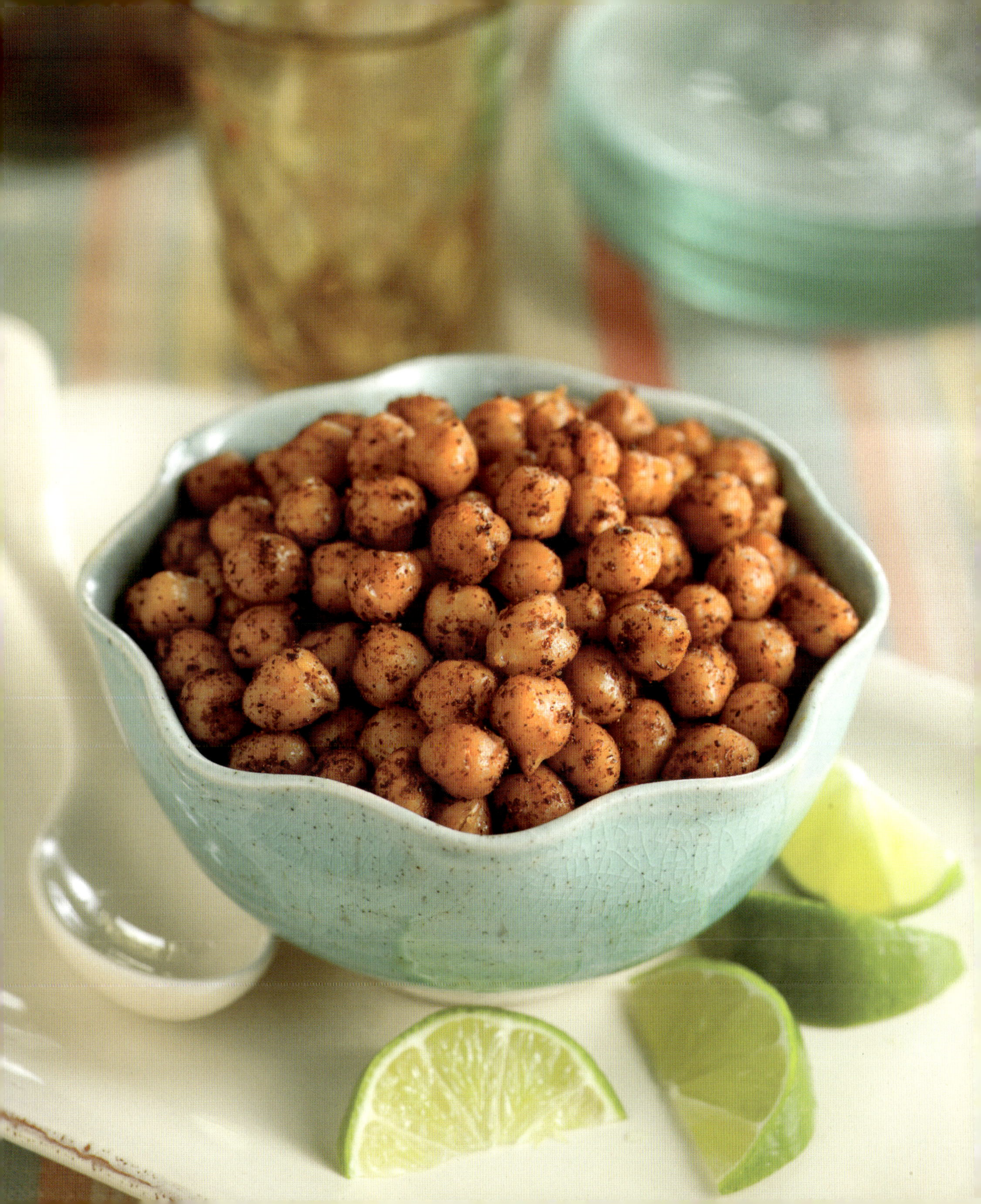

Fruit Kabobs with Raspberry Yogurt Dip

makes 6 servings

- ½ cup plain nonfat Greek yogurt
- ¼ cup no-sugar-added raspberry fruit spread
- 1 pint fresh strawberries
- 2 cups cubed honeydew melon (1-inch cubes)
- 2 cups cubed cantaloupe (1-inch cubes)
- 1 cup fresh pineapple cubes

1. Stir yogurt and fruit spread in small bowl until well blended.
2. Thread fruit alternately onto six 12-inch skewers. Serve with yogurt dip.

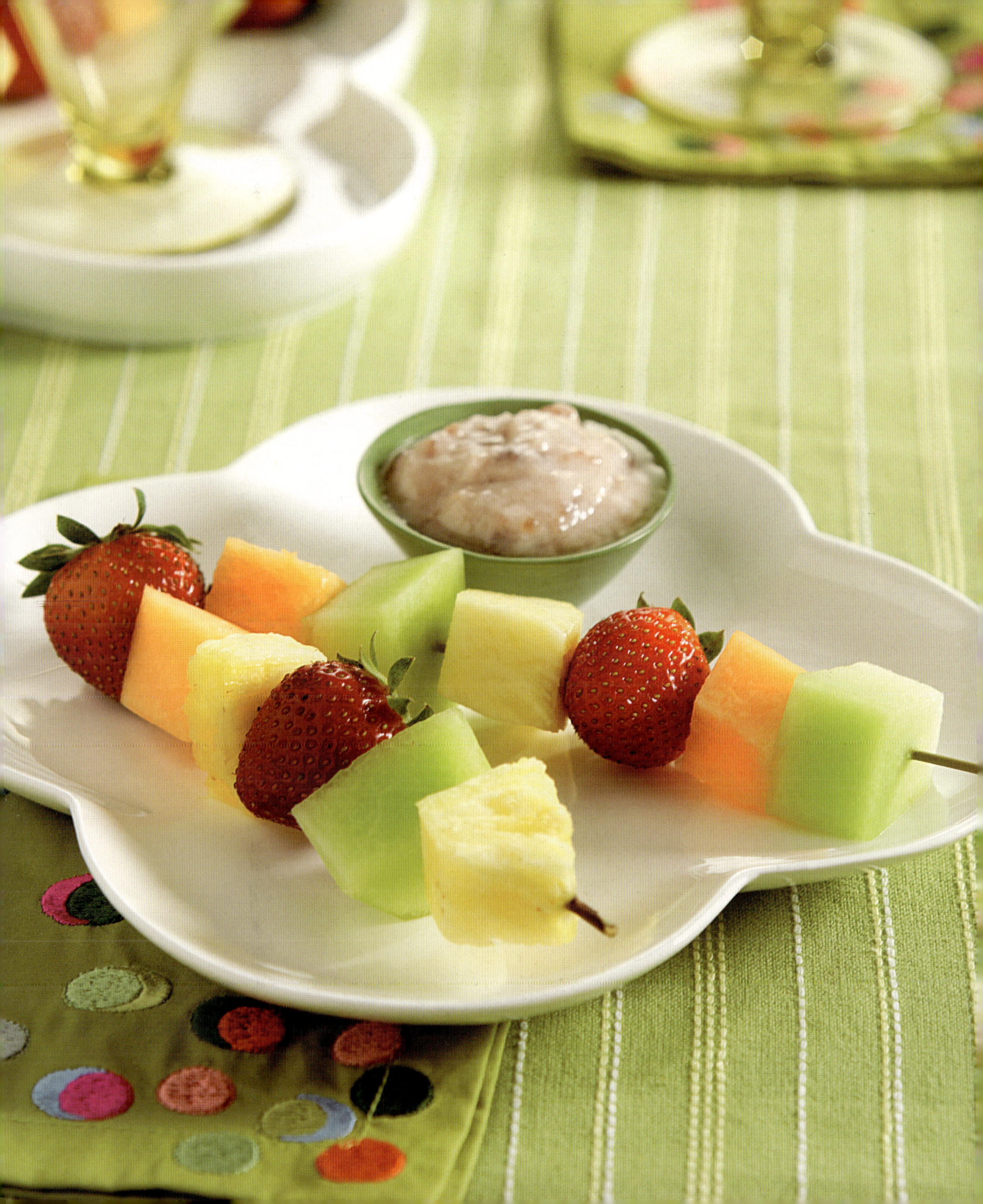

Chai Spiced Brown Rice and Chia Pudding

makes 4 to 6 servings

- **4 English breakfast tea bags**
- **½ cup uncooked short grain brown rice, rinsed well**
- **¼ cup chia seeds**
- **¼ teaspoon ground cardamom**
- **1 teaspoon ground cinnamon**
- **½ teaspoon ground ginger**
- **¼ teaspoon salt**
- **4 cups almond milk**
- **2 tablespoons maple syrup**
- **¼ cup raisins**

1. Pour 1 cup boiling water into glass measuring cup. Add tea bags; steep 5 minutes. Discard tea bags.
2. Combine tea, rice, chia seeds, cardamom, cinnamon, ginger, salt, milk and maple syrup in large saucepan; bring to a boil over medium-high heat. Reduce heat to low; partially cover and cook 1 hour 30 minutes or until rice is tender and mixture is thick and creamy, stirring occasionally.
3. Remove any film that appears on surface. Stir in raisins. Serve warm or at room temperature.

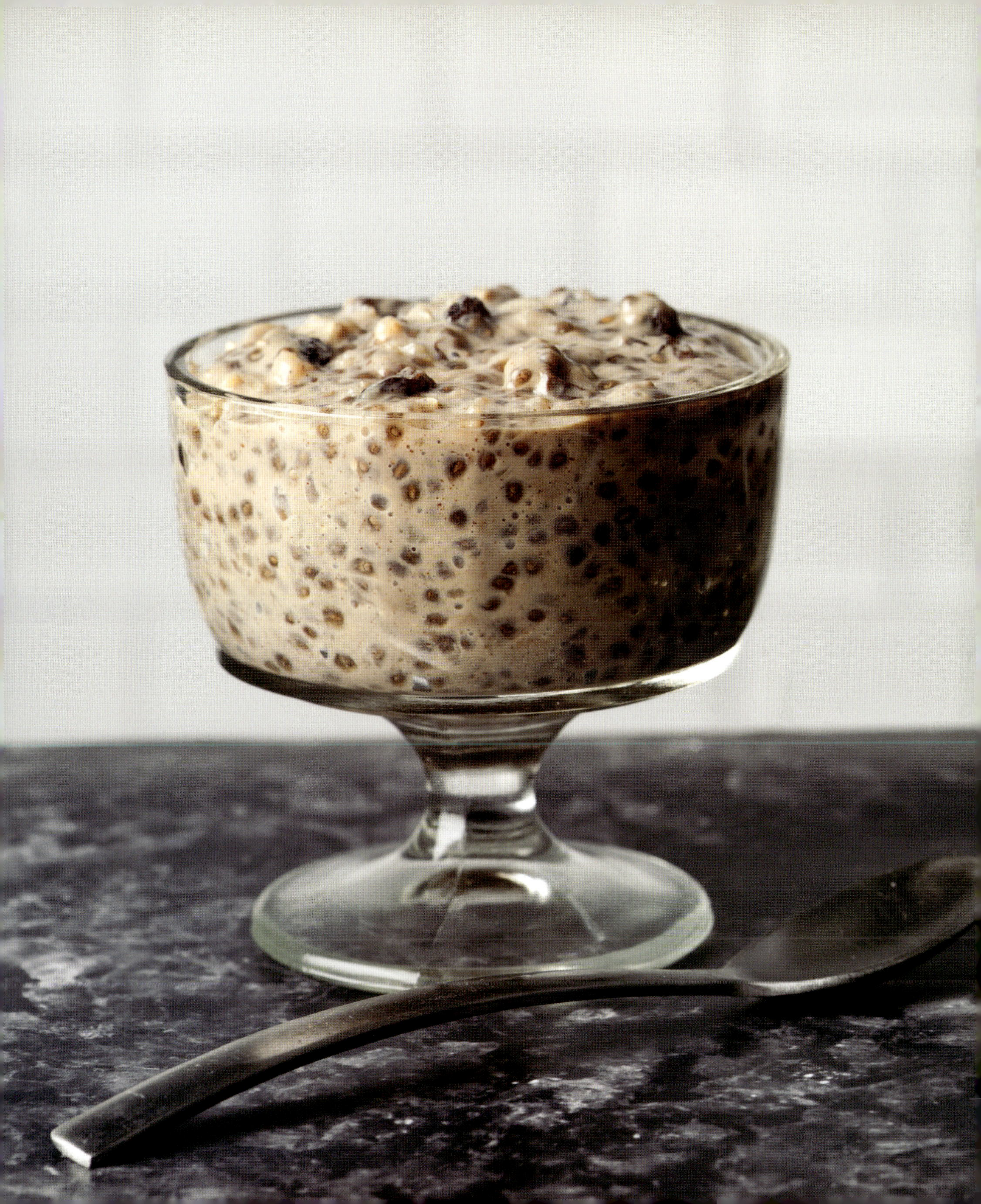

Chocolate Almond Truffles

makes 20 truffles (4 truffles per serving)

½ cup almond butter

3 tablespoons sugar substitute, such as stevia

1 cup crisp rice cereal

3 tablespoons unsweetened cocoa powder

¼ cup semisweet chocolate chips

1. Place almond butter in small microwavable bowl. Microwave on HIGH 10 seconds. Stir in sugar substitute with wooden spoon until smooth. Stir in cereal; mix well.
2. Line large plate with waxed paper. Spray hands with nonstick cooking spray and shape mixture into 1-inch balls, pressing firmly. Place balls on prepared plate and freeze 15 minutes or up to 1 hour.
3. Spread cocoa on small plate. Roll each truffle in cocoa; return to large plate.
4. Place chocolate chips in small resealable food storage bag. Microwave on HIGH 10 seconds; knead bag. Repeat until chocolate is melted and smooth.
5. Press melted chocolate into one corner of bag; cut small hole in corner. Drizzle chocolate over truffles; let stand until chocolate is set. Truffles can be refrigerated in airtight container up to 3 days.

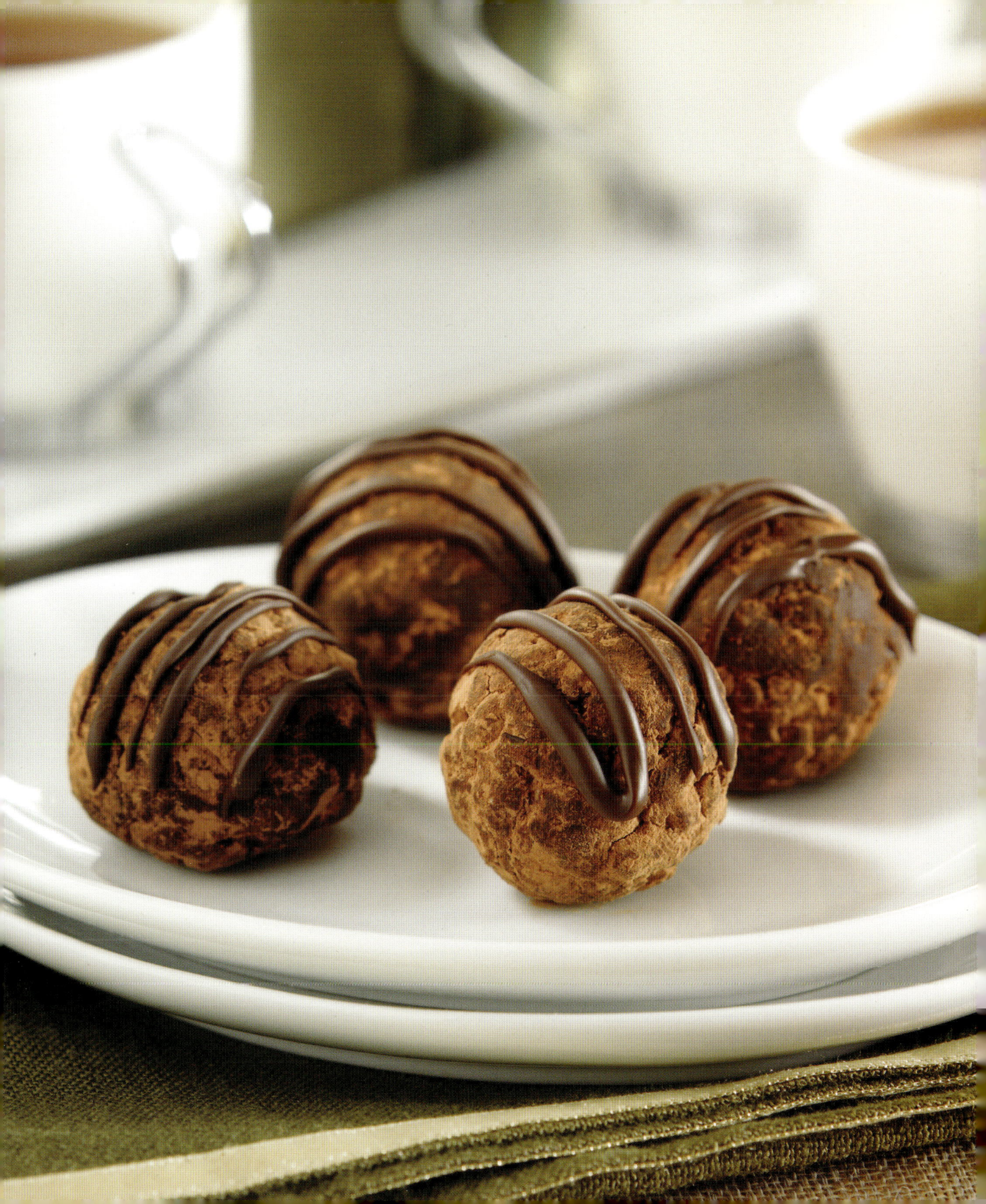

Banana Chocolate Chip Pops

makes 4 servings

- 1 small ripe banana
- 1 container (6 ounces) plain nonfat Greek yogurt
- ⅛ teaspoon ground nutmeg
- 2 tablespoons semi-sweet chocolate chips
- 4 pop molds or paper cups and pop sticks

1. Slice banana; place in food processor. Add yogurt and nutmeg; process until smooth. Transfer to small bowl; stir in chocolate chips.
2. Spoon banana mixture into molds or cups. Set on level surface in freezer; freeze 2 hours or until firm.
3. To unmold, briefly run warm water over molds until each pop loosens.

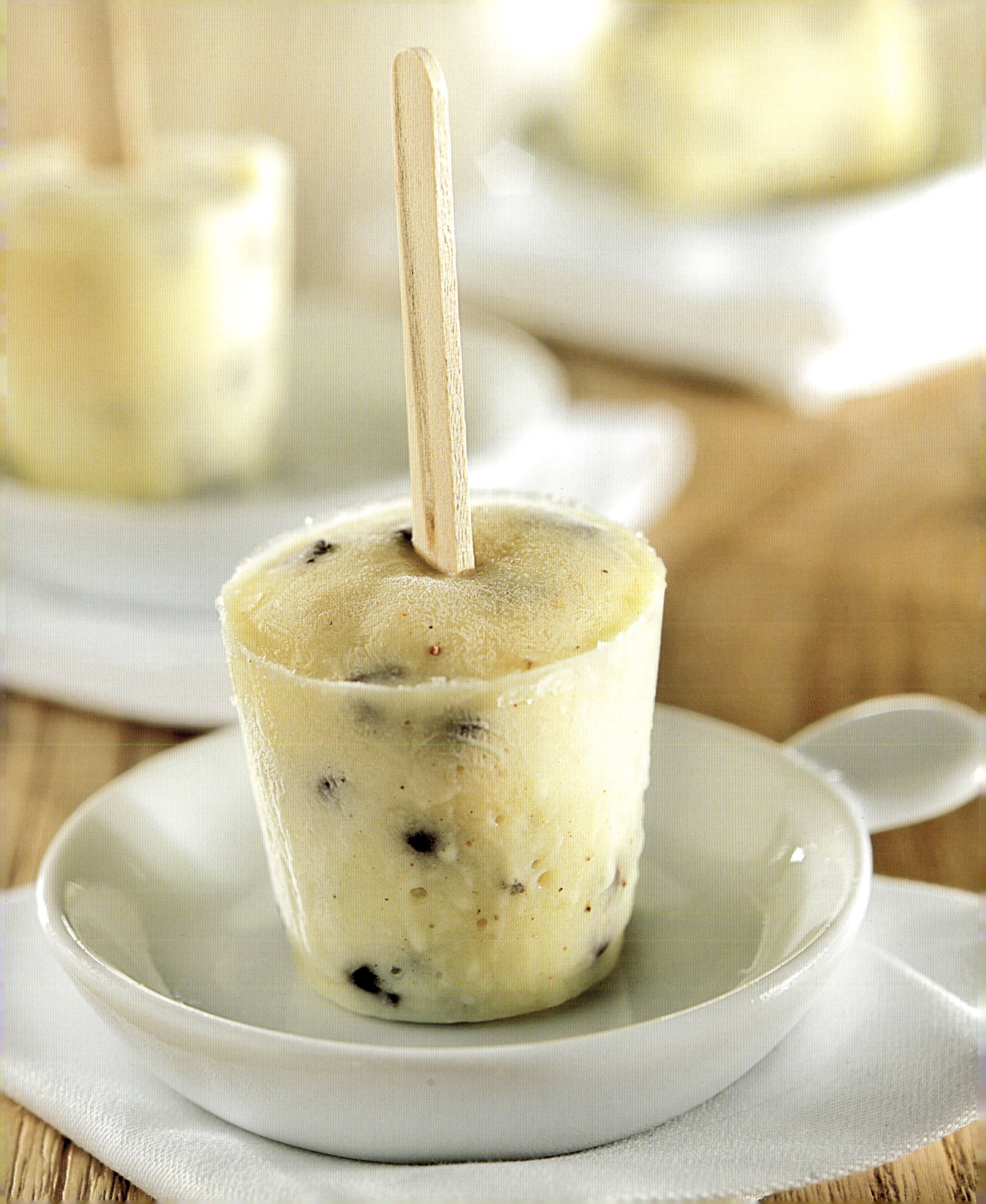

INDEX

Metric Conversion Chart

VOLUME MEASUREMENTS (dry)

1/8 teaspoon = 0.5 mL
1/4 teaspoon = 1 mL
1/2 teaspoon = 2 mL
3/4 teaspoon = 4 mL
1 teaspoon = 5 mL
1 tablespoon = 15 mL
2 tablespoons = 30 mL
1/4 cup = 60 mL
1/3 cup = 75 mL
1/2 cup = 125 mL
2/3 cup = 150 mL
3/4 cup = 175 mL
1 cup = 250 mL
2 cups = 1 pint = 500 mL
3 cups = 750 mL
4 cups = 1 quart = 1 L

VOLUME MEASUREMENTS (fluid)

1 fluid ounce (2 tablespoons) = 30 mL
4 fluid ounces (1/2 cup) = 125 mL
8 fluid ounces (1 cup) = 250 mL
12 fluid ounces (1 1/2 cups) = 375 mL
16 fluid ounces (2 cups) = 500 mL

WEIGHTS (mass)

1/2 ounce = 15 g
1 ounce = 30 g
3 ounces = 90 g
4 ounces = 120 g
8 ounces = 225 g
10 ounces = 285 g
12 ounces = 360 g
16 ounces = 1 pound = 450 g

DIMENSIONS

1/16 inch = 2 mm
1/8 inch = 3 mm
1/4 inch = 6 mm
1/2 inch = 1.5 cm
3/4 inch = 2 cm
1 inch = 2.5 cm

OVEN TEMPERATURES

250°F = 120°C
275°F = 140°C
300°F = 150°C
325°F = 160°C
350°F = 180°C
375°F = 190°C
400°F = 200°C
425°F = 220°C
450°F = 230°C

BAKING PAN SIZES

Utensil	Size in Inches/Quarts	Metric Volume	Size in Centimeters
Baking or Cake Pan (square or rectangular)	8×8×2	2 L	20×20×5
	9×9×2	2.5 L	23×23×5
	12×8×2	3 L	30×20×5
	13×9×2	3.5 L	33×23×5
Loaf Pan	8×4×3	1.5 L	20×10×7
	9×5×3	2 L	23×13×7
Round Layer Cake Pan	8×1½	1.2 L	20×4
	9×1½	1.5 L	23×4
Pie Plate	8×1¼	750 mL	20×3
	9×1¼	1 L	23×3
Baking Dish or Casserole	1 quart	1 L	—
	1½ quart	1.5 L	—
	2 quart	2 L	—

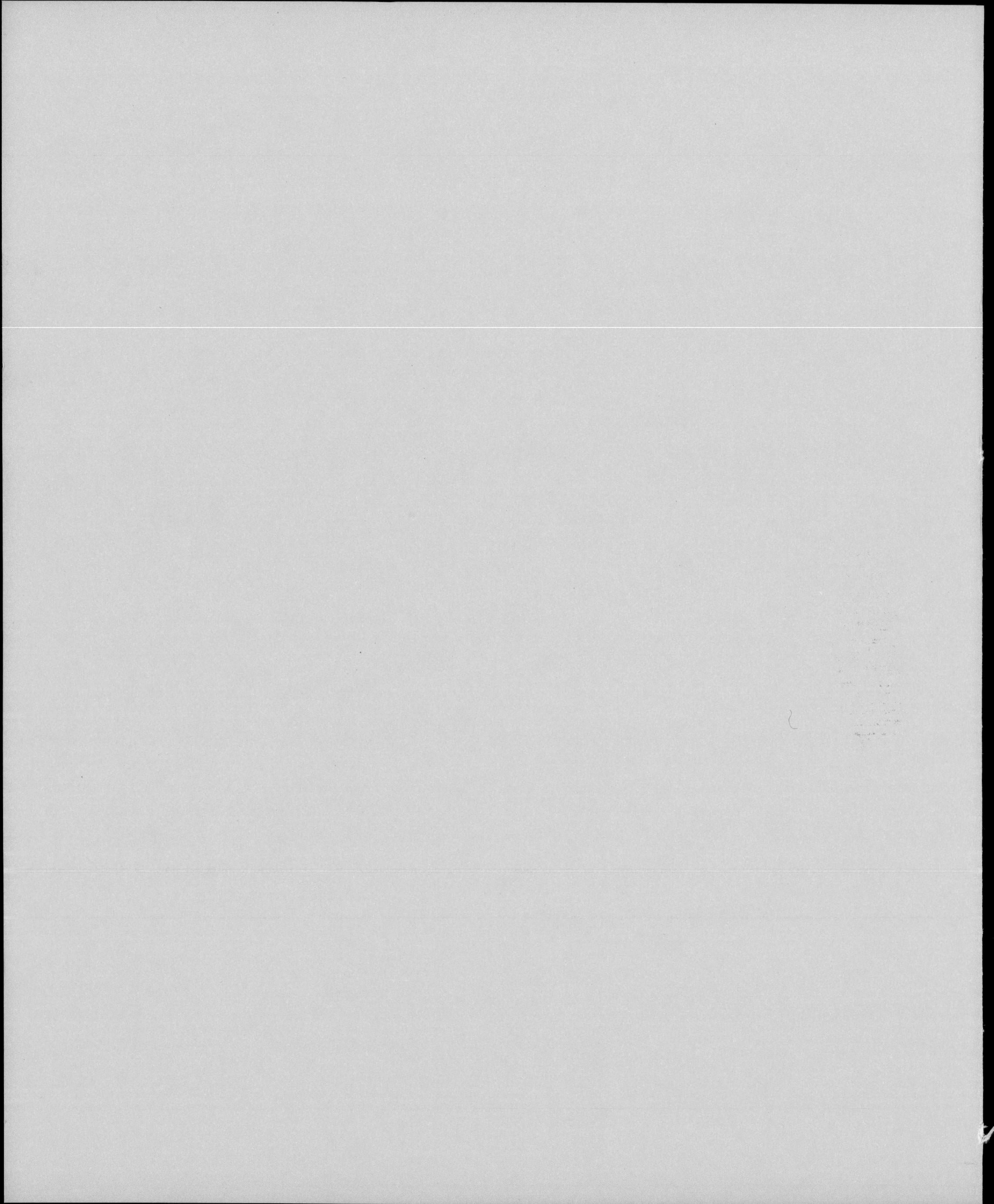